Handb
Endocrinology

Rajesh K. Garg
James V. Hennessey
Alan Ona Malabanan
Jeffrey R. Garber
Editors

Handbook of Inpatient Endocrinology

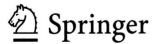 Springer

Editors
Rajesh K. Garg
Division of Endocrinology
Diabetes and Metabolism
University of Miami Miller
School of Medicine
Coral Gables
FL
USA

Alan Ona Malabanan
Beth Israel Deaconess
Medical Center
Harvard Medical School
Division of Endocrinology
Diabetes and Metabolism
Boston
MA
USA

James V. Hennessey
Beth Israel Deaconess
Medical Center
Harvard Medical School
Division of Endocrinology
Diabetes and Metabolism
Boston
MA
USA

Jeffrey R. Garber
Beth Israel Deaconess
Medical Center
Brigham and Women's Hospital
Harvard Medical School
Department of Endocrinology
Boston
MA
USA

ISBN 978-3-030-38975-8   ISBN 978-3-030-38976-5   (eBook)
https://doi.org/10.1007/978-3-030-38976-5

This Springer imprint is published by the registered company Springer Nature Switzerland AG
The registered company address is: Gewerbestrasse 11, 6330 Cham, Switzerland

Dedicated to our fellows.

– Rajesh K. Garg,
James V. Hennessey,
Alan Ona Malabanan,
and Jeffrey R. Garber

Preface

During the last two decades, there has been increasing emphasis on physicians seeing more patients in ambulatory settings. As a result, hospital-based physicians are providing more inpatient care, and fewer endocrinologists, after fellowship training, are caring for their hospitalized patients. Yet managing endocrine diseases in the inpatient setting has become more complex, while transitioning that care back to the ambulatory setting is as critical as ever. Examples of complex care and challenges regularly encountered in hospitalized patients abound and include managing diabetes emergencies, those with diabetes mellitus on total parenteral nutrition, insulin treatment protocols for pregnancy in diabetes, and thyroid crises. Additionally, the diagnosis and management of adrenal insufficiency; perioperative care of patients undergoing pituitary, parathyroid, adrenal, and thyroid surgery; and patients with thyroid dysfunction who have heart disease as well as those who cannot take oral medications frequently are encountered. The editors of this handbook, attending endocrinologists in Boston's Longwood Medical Area at either the Brigham and Women's Hospital or Beth Israel Medical Center, decided to produce this volume after agreeing that even the most experienced endocrinologist working on a busy inpatient consult service would benefit from an easy-to-navigate and concise text for guidance.

Many authors were in their fellowship training when they contributed to this book. The book is designed to highlight salient clinical points with more detailed information available on each point. The well-established clinical approaches are emphasized with suggestions for further reading. In addition to serving as a practical, easy-to-navigate reference guide for those taking care of inpatients with endocrine disorders, each section provides guidance about bridging their care from the inpatient to the outpatient setting.

The audience for this book includes physicians who provide most inpatient consultative care, for example, endocrinology fellows, their attending physicians, surgical and obstetrical specialists, primary care physicians, and hospitalists. We look forward to receiving your feedback so that future editions can remain up-to-date and we can address issues that we have not sufficiently emphasized in this, our first edition.

Coral Gables, FL, USA   Rajesh K. Garg
Boston, MA, USA   James V. Hennessey
                                                         Alan Ona Malabanan
                                                           Jeffrey R. Garber

Contents

Contributors

Ana Paula Abreu, MD, PhD Division of Endocrinology, Diabetes and Hypertension, Department of Medicine, Brigham and Women's Hospital and Harvard Medical School, Boston, MA, USA

Trevor E. Angell, MD Keck School of Medicine, University of Southern California, Division of Endocrinology and Diabetes, Los Angeles, CA, USA

Alejandro Raul Ayala, MD University of Miami, Miller School of Medicine, Department of Endocrinology and Metabolism, Miami, FL, USA

Florence M. Brown, MD Joslin-Beth Israel Deaconess Medical Center Diabetes in Pregnancy Program, Joslin Diabetes Center, Department of Adult Diabetes, Boston, MA, USA

Hsin-Yun Chang, MD National Cheng Kung University Hospital, Department of Family Medicine, Tainan City, Taiwan

Marcy A. Cheifetz, MD Harvard Vanguard Medical Associates, Atrius Health, Department of Endocrinology, Chestnut Hill, MA, USA

Zsu-Zsu Chen, MD Beth Israel Deaconess Medical Center, Department of Endocrinology, Diabetes and Metabolism, Boston, MA, USA

Bradley M. Denker, MD Beth Israel Deaconess Medical Center, Department of Medicine, Nephrology Division and Harvard Medical School, Boston, MA, USA

Erika R. Drury, MD Division of Nephrology, Department of Medicine, University of Rochester School of Medicine, Rochester, NY, USA

Anna Zelfond Feldman, MD Harvard Medical School, Beth Israel Deaconess Medical Center, Department of Endocrinology, Boston, MA, USA

Brandon P. Galm, MD, MPH, FRCPC Neuroendocrine Unit, Massachusetts General Hospital and Harvard Medical School, Boston, MA, USA

Om P. Ganda, MD Joslin Diabetes Center, Department of Medicine, Beth Israel Deaconess Medical Center, Boston, MA, USA

Jeffrey R. Garber, MD Beth Israel Deaconess Medical Center, Brigham and Women's Hospital, Harvard Medical School, Department of Endocrinology, Boston, MA, USA

Rajesh K. Garg, MD Division of Endocrinology, Diabetes and Metabolism, University of Miami Miller School of Medicine, Coral Gables, FL, USA

Ole-Petter R. Hamnvik, MB BCh BAO, Mmsc, MRCPI Brigham and Women's Hospital, Department of Medicine, Division of Endocrinology, Diabetes and Hypertension, Boston, MA, USA

Pamela Hartzband, MD Harvard Medical School, Beth Israel Deaconess Medical Center, Department of Endocrinology and Metabolism, Boston, MA, USA

James V. Hennessey, MD Beth Israel Deaconess Medical Center, Harvard Medical School, Division of Endocrinology, Diabetes and Metabolism, Boston, MA, USA

Margo Hudson, MD Brigham and Women's Hospital, Department of Endocrinology, Hypertension and Diabetes, Boston, MA, USA

Gwendolyne Anyanate Jack, MD, MPH Weill Cornell Medical Center-New York Presbyterian Hospital, Department of Medicine, Division of Endocrinology, Diabetes and Metabolism, New York, NY, USA

Mark Anthony Jara, MD University of Miami, Miller School of Medicine, Division of Endocrinology and Metabolism, Miami, FL, USA

Ursula B. Kaiser, MD Division of Endocrinology, Diabetes and Hypertension, Department of Medicine, Brigham and Women's Hospital and Harvard Medical School, Boston, MA, USA

Melissa G. Lechner, MD, PhD David Geffen School of Medicine, University of California at Los Angeles, Division of Endocrinology, Diabetes and Metabolism, Los Angeles, CA, USA

Alan Ona Malabanan, MD, FACE, CCD Beth Israel Deaconess Medical Center, Harvard Medical School, Division of Endocrinology, Diabetes and Metabolism, Boston, MA, USA

Roselyn Cristelle I. Mateo, MD MSc Joslin Diabetes Center, Department of Endocrinology, Beth Israel Deaconess Medical Center, Boston, MA, USA

J. Carl Pallais, MD, MPH Brigham and Women's Hospital, Division of Endocrinology, Department of Medicine, Boston, MA, USA

Johanna A. Pallotta, MD Harvard Medical School, Beth Israel Deaconess Medical Center, Department of Medicine, Endocrinology and Metabolism, Boston, MA, USA

Daniela V. Pirela, MD Jackson Memorial Hospital/University of Miami Hospital, Division of Endocrinology, Diabetes and Metabolism, Miami, FL, USA

Megan Ritter, MD Weill Cornell Medicine, New York Presbyterian, New York, NY, USA

Jeena Sandeep, MD St. Elizabeth Medical Center, Department of Medicine, Division of Endocrinology, Brighton, MA, USA

Julian L. Seifter, MD Brigham and Women's Hospital, Department of Medicine, Boston, MA, USA

Antonia E. Stephen, MD Harvard Medical School, Massachusetts General Hospital, Department of Surgery, Boston, MA, USA

Catherine J. Tang, MD Beth Israel Deaconess Medical Center, Harvard Medical School, Division of Endocrinology, Diabetes and Metabolism, Boston, MA, USA

Elena Toschi, MD Adult Clinic, Joslin Diabetes Center, Harvard Medical School, Beth Israel Deaconess Medical Center, Department of Endocrinology and Diabetes, Boston, MA, USA

Nicholas A. Tritos, MD, DSc Harvard Medical School, Massachusetts General Hospital, Neuroendocrine Unit and Neuroendocrine & Pituitary Tumor Clinical Center, Boston, MA, USA

Anand Vaidya, MD, MMSc Harvard Medical School, Center for Adrenal Disorders, Division of Endocrinology, Diabetes, and Hypertension, Brigham and Women's Hospital, Boston, MA, USA

Maria Vamvini, MD Adult Clinic, Joslin Diabetes Center, Harvard Medical School, Beth Israel Deaconess Medical Center, Department of Endocrinology and Diabetes, Boston, MA, USA

Gregory P. Westcott, MD Beth Israel Deaconess Medical Center and Joslin Diabetes Center, Department of Endocrinology, Diabetes and Metabolism, Boston, MA, USA

Pituitary Apoplexy

1

Ana Paula Abreu and Ursula B. Kaiser

Contents

A. P. Abreu (✉) · U. B. Kaiser
Division of Endocrinology, Diabetes and Hypertension, Department of
Medicine, Brigham and Women's Hospital and Harvard Medical School,
Boston, MA, USA
e-mail: apabreu@bwh.harvard.edu; ukaiser@bwh.harvard.edu

© Springer Nature Switzerland AG 2020
R. K. Garg et al. (eds.), *Handbook of Inpatient Endocrinology*,
https://doi.org/10.1007/978-3-030-38976-5_1

Definition

Apoplexy means "sudden attack" in Greek. Classical pituitary apoplexy (PA) is a clinical syndrome characterized by abrupt hemorrhage and/or infarction of the pituitary gland. Severe headache of sudden onset is the main symptom, sometimes associated with visual disturbances or ocular palsy. Apoplexy usually occurs in patients with preexisting pituitary adenomas and evolves within hours or days.

Subclinical PA is defined as asymptomatic or unrecognized pituitary hemorrhage and/or infarction. It may be detected on routine imaging or during histopathological examination. The frequency of subclinical hemorrhagic infarction in pituitary tumors is around 25%.

Precipitating Factors/Patients at Risk

The precise pathophysiology of PA is not completely understood. Since most cases occur in preexisting pituitary adenomas, it has been hypothesized that a reduction in blood flow or abnormal vascularity of the tumor could be mechanisms contributing to PA. The underlying process can be simple infarction, hemorrhagic infarction, or mixed hemorrhagic infarction.

The pituitary gland is enlarged in pregnancy and prone to infarction from hypovolemic shock. Pituitary necrosis that occurs in the setting of large-volume obstetric hemorrhage postpartum is referred to as Sheehan syndrome. It is a rare but potentially life-threatening complication that can result in postpartum hypopituitarism.

The clinical symptoms of PA mimic other common neurological disorders such as subarachnoid hemorrhage, migraine, bacterial meningitis, or stroke, which can lead to delayed or even missed diagnosis. A high degree of clinical suspicion is needed to diagnose pituitary apoplexy, as most patients do not have a previous history of known pituitary adenoma. Precipitating risk factors have been identified in 10–40% of cases of PA, and it is important to recognize them. Hypertension has been considered a precipitating factor for PA, although recent studies question this association. Surgery, particularly coronary artery surgery, and angiographic procedures have been reported to be associated with PA. Dynamic testing of pituitary function, using growth hormone-releasing hormone, gonadotropin-releasing hormone, thyrotropin-releasing hormone, and corticotrophin-releasing hormone (less commonly), or an insulin tolerance test, is also associated with PA. Initiation or withdrawal of dopamine receptor agonists, estrogen therapy, radiation therapy, pregnancy, head trauma, and coagulopathy are some other factors known to induce pituitary apoplexy. A diagnosis of PA should be considered in all patients with these risk factors who present with acute severe headache, with or without neuro-ophthalmologic signs.

Diagnosis

Obtain Detailed Clinical History

The clinical presentation can be acute or subacute and is highly variable, determined by the extent of hemorrhage, necrosis, and edema. Headache is present in more than 80% of patients. It is usually retro-orbital but can be bifrontal or diffuse. Nausea and vomiting can be associated. As most patients have an underlying macroadenoma, signs and symptoms of hypopituitarism may have been present prior to the episode of PA. As discussed earlier, most patients do not have a history of a known prior pituitary adenoma and therefore do not carry a diagnosis of hypopituitarism.

Sheehan syndrome usually presents with a combination of failure to lactate postdelivery and amenorrhea or oligomenorrhea, but any of the manifestations of hypopituitarism (e.g., hypotension, hyponatremia, hypothyroidism) can occur at any time from the immediate postpartum period to years after delivery.

Perform Detailed Physical Exam Including Cranial Nerves and Visual Fields

More than half of patients with PA have some degree of visual field impairment, with bitemporal hemianopsia being the most common. About half of patients have oculomotor palsies due to functional impairment of cranial nerves III, IV, and/or VI. Cranial nerve III is most commonly affected, resulting in ptosis, limited eye adduction, and mydriasis due to nerve compression. Extravasation of blood or necrotic tissue into the subarachnoid space can result in meningismus and an altered level of consciousness.

Evaluation of Endocrine Dysfunction/Laboratory Assessment

Most patients will have dysfunction of one or more pituitary hormones at the time of initial presentation. The most clinically important hormone deficiency is adrenocorticotrophic hormone (ACTH), which can be life-threatening. It is present in 50–80% of patients and can cause hemodynamic instability and hyponatremia. Of note, hyponatremia is a consequence of cortisol deficiency, with loss of feedback inhibition of arginine vasopressin/antidiuretic hormone (ADH) release despite hypoosmolality and a direct water excretion defect. Additionally, hypothalamic irritation in the setting of PA can result in the syndrome of inappropriate antidiuretic hormone. Nausea/vomiting and hypoglycemia (secondary to GH and/or ACTH deficiency) are also stimuli for ADH secretion. Secondary hypothyroidism can also contribute to hyponatremia.

Patients with suspected PA should have electrolytes, renal function, kidney function, coagulation, and CBC checked to assess for risk factors and for the general condition of the patient.

Pituitary endocrine evaluation is necessary to diagnose secretory pituitary adenomas as well as hypopituitarism. An initial random cortisol, ACTH, LH, FSH, testosterone or estradiol, FT4, TSH, IGF-1, and prolactin should be measured immediately upon the diagnosis of PA to screen for a hyperfunctioning pituitary adenoma. Low serum prolactin at presentation is seen in patients with the highest intrasellar pressure, who are less likely to recover pituitary function. It is important to emphasize that blood samples for ACTH and cortisol measurements should be obtained prior to the administration of steroids. The hypothalamic-pituitary-adrenal axis usually responds to critical illness with an increase in serum cortisol levels, and it is expected that a random cortisol level will similarly be elevated during the acute phase of PA without hypopituitarism. There is no clearly agreed-upon cut-off for random cortisol levels for the diagnosis of adrenal insufficiency during the acute phase of PA, but studies have shown that in patients with PA and proven central adrenal insufficiency, cortisol levels are very low.

Approximately 40–70% of patients with PA have thyrotropin or gonadotropin deficiency. Hormone replacement of these deficiencies can begin when the patient has recovered from the acute illness. GH deficiency is seen in almost all patients but is not always tested or treated.

Diabetes insipidus is present in less than 5% of patients with PA and may be further masked by the development of secondary adrenal failure and/or hypothyroidism.

Imaging

CT is usually the initial imaging modality performed for patients with sudden onset of headache. CT is useful to rule out subarachnoid hemorrhage and can detect a sellar mass in up to 80% of cases. In 20–30% of cases, the CT scan will detect hemorrhage into the pituitary mass, confirming the diagnosis of PA. Magnetic resonance imaging (MRI) is the imaging procedure of choice and has been found to identify an underlying tumor, if present, in over 90% of the cases. Therefore, MRI is more sensitive for the diagnosis of PA and should be done in all patients with suspected

PA. MRI can detect hemorrhagic and necrotic areas and can show the relationship between a tumor and adjacent structures such as the optic chiasm, cavernous sinus, and hypothalamus (Fig. 1.1). However, conventional MRI sequences may not detect an infarct

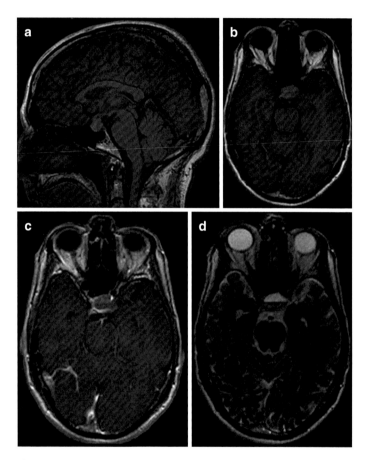

Fig. 1.1 MRI of a patient with pituitary apoplexy. Images were obtained approximately 24 hours after onset of symptoms (sudden headache, nausea, vomiting, and fatigue). Images show enlargement of the pituitary gland, which contains a fluid hematocrit level. (**a**) T1 sagittal, the upper margin of the pituitary gland is contacting and slightly displacing the optic chiasm superiorly. (**b**) Axial pre-contrast. (**c**) T1 axial post gadolinium. (**d**) T2 axial

for up to 6 hours after the acute event. Diffusion-weighted imaging (DWI) is a commonly performed MRI sequence for the detection of small infarcts and initial hemorrhage and can be very helpful in the early phases of PA.

Thickening of the sphenoid mucosa in the sphenoid sinus beneath the sella turcica has been reported during the acute phase of PA and corresponds with marked mucosal swelling from increased pressure in the venous sinuses draining the sinus area. Such mucosal thickening has been shown to correlate with worse neurological and endocrinological outcomes.

Management

Patients with PA should be managed by neurosurgeons and endocrinologists in a hospital with an acute care neurosurgical unit available and with access to ophthalmological evaluation.

Consider Initiation of Corticosteroid Treatment

PA can be a true medical emergency. The course of PA is variable and management will depend on a patient's clinical condition. The first intervention is hemodynamic stabilization and correction of electrolyte disturbances. As corticotropin deficiency is present in the vast majority of patients and may be life-threatening, corticosteroids should be administered intravenously as soon as the diagnosis is confirmed and blood is collected for cortisol and ACTH measurement. A bolus of 100 mg (some studies recommend 200 mg) of hydrocortisone followed by 50–100 mg IV every 6–8 hours is given; alternatively, 2–4 mg/h by continuous administration should be given. There are no randomized trials comparing different doses, so the ideal dose of hydrocortisone administration is not known. Dexamethasone may be used instead of hydrocortisone to reduce edema as a part of a conservative approach for treatment of PA. Although the majority of the literature recommends empiric corticosteroid treatment for all patients with diagnosis of PA, the UK guidelines for the management of pituitary apoplexy recommend steroid therapy in patients with hemodynamic instability, altered level of consciousness, reduced visual acuity, and severe visual field defects, or if a 9:00 am cortisol is less than 18 mcg/dL.

Acute Intervention: Surgery vs. Conservative Treatment

Most cases of PA improve with either surgical or expectant management, but the most appropriate approach in the acute phase is controversial. Studies comparing the two modalities are retrospective and suffer from selection bias. The ideal surgical treatment is via the transsphenoidal approach. One important factor to consider is the risk of surgery, and in the acute setting, the operation may be performed by the on-call neurosurgeon rather than by skilled pituitary surgeons; this may increase the risk of complications. Studies suggest that the posttreatment prevalence of pituitary deficiency is similar after either treatment modality. The endocrine prognosis is poorer in patients with pituitary adenoma and PA than in uncomplicated pituitary adenoma, as pituitary damage more commonly occurs during the acute apoplectic event. Studies suggest that visual field defects improve or normalize in most patients regardless of the treatment modality. However, it is the general consensus – and is the recommendation by the UK guidelines for the management of PA – to consider surgical treatment in patients with severe neuro-ophthalmologic signs such as severely reduced visual acuity or severe and persistent or deteriorating visual field defects. A deteriorating level of consciousness is also an indication for surgical treatment. Studies suggest, although one should keep selection bias in mind, that patients treated conservatively have better outcomes with regard to ocular palsies. Resolution of ocular paresis resulting from involvement of cranial nerve III, IV, or VI is usually seen within days to weeks, and it is not an indication for surgery. Surgery should be performed within 7 days of the onset of the symptoms. One study showed that the prognosis of visual defects is less favorable when surgery is done more than a week after onset. A Pituitary Apoplexy

Table 1.1 Pituitary Apoplexy Score

Variable	Points
Level of consciousness	
Glasgow Coma Scale 15	0
Glasgow Coma Scale 8–14	2
Glasgow Coma Scale <8	4
Visual acuity	
Normal	0
Reduced unilateral	1
Reduced bilateral	2
Visual field defects	
Normal	0
Unilateral defect	1
Bilateral defect	2
Ocular paresis	
Absent	0
Present unilateral	1
Present bilateral	2

Reprinted with permission from Rajasekaran S, Vanderpump M, Baldeweg S, et al. UK guidelines for the management of pituitary apoplexy. Clin Endocrinol;74(1):9–20, © 2011, with permission from John Wiley and Sons

Score (see Table 1.1) was designed by the UK guidelines for the management of PA to enable more uniform clinical description of PA and enable better comparison between different management options.

It is rare to change from conservative treatment to an operative course, but urgent imaging should be done in the presence of a new or deteriorating visual field deficit or neurological deterioration.

Reduction in tumor size is frequent after apoplexy, and follow-up imaging can show empty sella, partially empty sella, or even normal pituitary. The tumor recurrence rate is similar with both treatment modalities, and it has been shown to be approximately 6%. Therefore, long-term surveillance is recommended. Patients with simple infarction on MRI typically have less severe clinical features and better outcomes than those with hemorrhage or hemorrhagic infarction.

Postoperative Care

Postoperative management of patients following surgery for PA is similar to that of elective pituitary surgery for pituitary tumors. In some cases, patients may not have had a complete evaluation prior to surgery, and the pituitary function status will not be known. An early postoperative CT or sellar MRI should be performed in any patient with a new or worsened neurological deficit such as visual deterioration or diplopia and in anyone with significant rhinorrhea and a suspected CSF leak.

Monitor for Signs and Laboratory Abnormalities Suggestive of Diabetes Insipidus (DI)

Alterations in sodium and fluid balance are relatively common in the early postoperative phase. The classic reported triphasic response, in which patients initially develop DI in the first 24 to 48 hours, followed by transient SIADH developing 4–10 days postoperatively, followed by the return of DI in a matter of weeks, is not the most common pattern seen postpituitary surgery but can occur. More often, patients present with DI within the first days postsurgery and then either recover completely or develop SIADH about 5 days postsurgery or later. Fluid balance, serum electrolytes, urea, creatinine, and plasma and urine osmolality should be monitored closely during the first week postsurgery. During the first 2 days after surgery, fluid balance, electrolytes, and urine and serum osmolality should be checked every 8–12 hours; thereafter, further monitoring will depend on the patient's clinical status.

DI is present in about 5% of the patients after PA but can be seen in up to 25% of patients undergoing transsphenoidal pituitary surgery. In most cases, the patients may develop transient DI but do not require any therapy. They should be allowed to drink to thirst and their serum sodium should be monitored closely. When treatment is needed, desmopressin (DDAVP) should be given subcutaneously or intravenously (0.5–2 mcg every 24 hours as needed), or alternatively, an oral formulation can be given (often starting with 0.1–0.2 mg orally as a single evening dose, with doses up to 0.3 mg orally three times daily sometimes needed). Intranasal DDAVP is not generally used acutely in patients who have undergone transsphenoidal surgery until after the nose has healed and nasal congestion has improved. SIADH, when it occurs, usually presents 4 to 10 days postoperatively and can often be treated with fluid restriction and close monitoring.

Assess Pituitary Reserve

As discussed above, most of the patients will receive corticosteroid treatment during the acute phase of PA. The dose should be tapered to replacement doses when the patient is clinically stable. In patients without a previous diagnosis of adrenal insufficiency, a morning fasting cortisol should be checked on day 2 or 3 after surgery to assess residual postpituitary infarction and post-steroid treatment reserve after the acute event of PA and postoperatively. Hydrocortisone should be held for at least 24 hours prior to measuring cortisol levels. In patients with known and documented cortisol deficiency before surgery, a morning cortisol level should be checked within 4 to 8 weeks to determine if they will need long-term steroid treatment.

TSH and free T4 (FT4) should be checked on day 3 or 4 postoperatively, and thyroid hormone replacement should be considered if deficient. The interpretation of thyroid function tests postsurgically should be careful as "sick euthyroid syndrome" can alter TSH and FT4 hormone levels and affect the interpretation of these tests. Thyroid deficiency may take several weeks to be diagnosed given thyroid gland reserve and the half-life of T4, so thyroid function can be normal in the immediate postoperative period; hence it is important to test it again ~4–8 weeks postoperatively or if symptoms of hypothyroidism develop.

Visual Assessment

Visual fields, eye movements, and visual acuity should be examined at the bedside as soon as the patient can cooperate with the examination, ideally within 48 hours. A formal visual field assessment using a Humphrey analyzer or Goldmann perimetry should be performed within a few weeks after the acute event.

Follow-Up After Discharge

Check Electrolytes After 1 Week

Patients should be seen in follow-up within 1 week of surgery to have sodium, thyroid function, ACTH, morning cortisol, and urine osmolality tested. As discussed earlier, patients may develop SIADH up to 10 days after surgery or after PA and should be monitored closely.

Reassess Pituitary Function After 4 to 8 Weeks

Hypopituitarism (discussed separately) is one of the complications of PA and may not be detected during the acute phase of PA. Thyroid deficiency may take several weeks to be diagnosed given thyroid gland reserve and T4 half-life. All patients should be seen 4–8 weeks after presenting with PA for evaluation of pituitary function. On the other hand, some pituitary hormonal deficiencies may recover postoperatively, and such recovery can also be assessed as part of this evaluation. Studies have shown partial or complete recovery of pituitary function in up to 50% of patients. In most cases, patients will be treated with glucocorticoids during the acute episode of PA; the long-term need for glucocorticoid replacement therapy should be determined at this time. Thyroid, adrenal, gonadal, and GH axes may be assessed at this visit. Patients should also have formal visual field, visual acuity, and eye movement assessment.

Patients treated for apoplexy should have at least annual biochemical assessment of pituitary function, which should usually include FT4, TSH, LH, FSH, testosterone in men, estradiol in women, prolactin, IGF-1, and dynamic tests of cortisol and growth hormone secretion if clinically appropriate.

Suggested Reading

Bonicki W, Kasperlik-Zaluska A, Koszewski W, Zgliczynski W, Wislawski J. Pituitary apoplexy: endocrine, surgical and oncological emergency. Incidence, clinical course and treatment with reference to 799 cases of pituitary adenomas. Acta Neurochir. 1993;120(3–4):118–22.

Briet C, Salenave S, Bonneville JF, Laws ER, Chanson P. Pituitary apoplexy. Endocr Rev. 2015;36(6):622–45. https://doi.org/10.1210/er.2015-1042.

Briet C, Salenave S, Chanson P. Pituitary apoplexy. Endocrinol Metab Clin N Am. 2015;44:199–209.

Loh JA, Verbalis JG. Diabetes insipidus as a complication after pituitary surgery. Nat Clin Pract Endocrinol Metab. 2007;3(6):489–94.

Rajasekaran S, Vanderpump M, Baldeweg S, et al. UK guidelines for the management of pituitary apoplexy. Clin Endocrinol. 2011;74:9–20.

Randeva HS, Schoebel J, Byrne J, Esiri M, Adams CB, Wass JA. Classical pituitary apoplexy: clinical features, management and outcome. Clin Endocrinol. 1999;51:181–8.

Semple PL, Jane JA Jr, Laws ER Jr. Clinical relevance of precipitating factors in pituitary apoplexy. Neurosurgery. 2007;61:956–61; discussion 61-2.

Sibal L, Ball SG, Connolly V, et al. Pituitary apoplexy: a review of clinical presentation, management and outcome in 45 cases. Pituitary. 2004;7:157–63.

Panhypopituitarism

2

Ana Paula Abreu and Ursula B. Kaiser

Contents

A. P. Abreu (✉) · U. B. Kaiser
Division of Endocrinology, Diabetes and Hypertension, Department of
Medicine, Brigham and Women's Hospital and Harvard Medical School,
Boston, MA, USA
e-mail: apabreu@bwh.harvard.edu; ukaiser@bwh.harvard.edu

© Springer Nature Switzerland AG 2020   15
R. K. Garg et al. (eds.), *Handbook of Inpatient Endocrinology*,
https://doi.org/10.1007/978-3-030-38976-5_2

Definition and Significance

Hypopituitarism is the inability of the pituitary gland to provide sufficient hormones for the needs of the individual. It is the result of the failure in either the production or secretion in one or more pituitary hormones. The diagnosis of hypopituitarism is important in the hospital because some hormone deficiencies, such as ACTH, pose significant risk to the patient's life and need to be treated. Also, it is crucial to diagnose and treat diabetes insipidus as it can cause hypernatremia, severe dehydration, coma, and death. The diagnosis of central hypothyroidism is challenging in the hospital, but thyroid hormone should be replaced in patients with secondary hypothyroidism. On the other hand, other pituitary hormone deficiencies do not pose acute risk to patient's life, and replacement may be postponed to the outpatient setting.

Identify Causes of Hypopituitarism

A high diagnostic suspicion is necessary to identify patients not previously diagnosed with hypopituitarism. Therefore, it is important to know what causes hypopituitarism in order to detect it (Table 2.1). Insults in the regulation, production, or secretion of any pituitary hormones can result in pituitary insufficiency. Physiological secretion of pituitary hormones relies on intact function of the hypothalamus.

Mass Lesions

Any structural disruption of the hypothalamic-pituitary region can cause decreased production or secretion of the hormones. Pituitary tumors are the most common cause of hypopituitarism, but any other tumor occupying the region can also cause pituitary dysfunction (Table 2.1). Mechanical compression of portal vessels and the

Table 2.1 Causes of hypopituitarism

Structural causes:	
Mass lesions	Pituitary adenoma Craniopharyngioma Rathke's cleft cyst Metastatic disease Lymphomas, germinomas, and other tumors
Infiltrative diseases	Hypophysitis (lymphocytic and others) Sarcoidosis Hemochromatosis Tuberculosis and other infections Syphilis
Vascular events	Pituitary apoplexy Sheehan's syndrome (infarction of the pituitary gland after postpartum hemorrhage) Intra-sellar carotid artery aneurysm
Traumatic injury	Traumatic brain injury Perinatal trauma Neurosurgery Radiation
Functional causes:	
Medications	Glucocorticoids Megestrol acetate Immunotherapy – CTLA-4 inhibitors/PDL1 antibodies Opioids GnRH agonists
Systemic diseases	Chronic illness Anorexia nervosa
Developmental and inherited genetic causes	Several genetic defects can cause isolated or combined pituitary deficiency

pituitary stalk, with resulting ischemic necrosis, is thought to be the predominant mechanism by which mass lesions cause hypopituitarism. Hyperprolactinemia in non-prolactin producing tumors is common with pituitary macroadenomas, given the disruption of the normal suppressive effects of dopamine from the hypothalamus.

Traumatic Brain Injury

This is an underestimated cause that can cause hypopituitarism even years after the trauma. Given the frequency of traumatic brain injury in the general population, it is important not to over-look this important cause of hypopituitarism.

Medications

Several medications can cause hypopituitarism. Chronic use of systemic corticosteroids inhibits the hypothalamic-pituitary-adrenal axis and is a common cause of central adrenal insuffi-ciency. This is very relevant for patients admitted to the hospital for acute disorders or for procedures, as they will need to receive higher doses of steroids (usually called stress doses of steroids) to compensate for the lack of an endogenous increase in the amount of cortisol production during stress. Chronic administration of some opioids such as fentanyl and hydromorphone has the poten-tial to cause secondary adrenal insufficiency as well as secondary hypogonadism. Immunotherapy causes hypopituitarism second-ary to hypophysitis that is discussed below.

Hypophysitis

Autoimmune hypophysitis and medication-induced hypophysitis can cause pituitary deficiency. Lymphocytic hypophysitis is more common in females, and more than half of the cases (57%) pres-ent during pregnancy or postpartum. Immunotherapy, used to treat melanoma, renal cell carcinoma, and other malignancies, can also cause hypophysitis. The pathophysiology and clinical pre-sentation of immunotherapy-induced hypophysitis are different from those of lymphocytic hypophysitis. The monoclonal anti-bodies, ipilimumab and tremelimumab, which bind and inhibit cytotoxic T-lymphocyte antigen-4 (CTLA-4), are reported to cause hypophysitis in 1–18% of treated patients. Most cases are caused by ipilimumab. The anti-programmed cell death protein antibodies (anti-PD-1 Abs), nivolumab and pembrolizumab, rarely cause hypophysitis. Patients with hypophysitis present with headache, pituitary enlargement, and hypopituitarism (Fig. 2.1). In most patients, the pituitary enlargement eventually resolves,

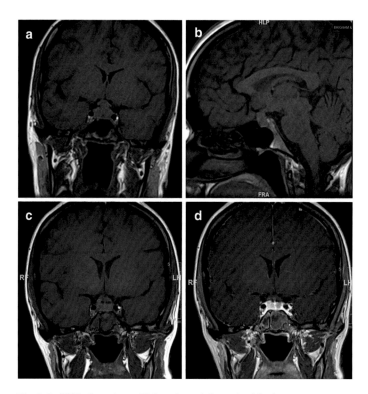

Fig. 2.1   MRI of a patient with lymphocytic hypophysitis. A pregnant woman presented to the emergency room at 30 weeks of gestational age with a 2-week history of worsening headaches and blurred vision in the last 24 hours: (**a**) coronal and (**b**) sagittal images without contrast showing enlargement of the pituitary gland, which measures approximately 1.4 cm in craniocaudal dimension. The gland has a convex superior border and is protruding into the suprasellar cistern. Since patient was pregnant, no contrast was given. Coronal images 3 months after the initial images and 1 month postpartum: (**c**) pre-gadolinium and (**d**) post-gadolinium. Images show interval decrease in size of anterior pituitary, which is no longer enlarged and now measures approximately 6 to 7 mm and demonstrates a flat superior surface

but hypopituitarism is usually permanent. The most common hormone deficiency in classical autoimmune lymphocytic hypophysitis is ACTH deficiency, seen in approximately 32% of the patients. Eighteen percent present with hyperprolactinemia and 31% develop diabetes insipidus. In anti-CTLA-4-induced hypophysitis, around 85% of the patients presented thyrotroph and gonadotroph deficiency, while 73% had corticotroph deficiency. In these cases, pituitary function recovered in approximately 25% of cases only.

Systemic Diseases

Infiltrative systemic diseases such as sarcoidosis, hemochromatosis, and rarely infiltrative infections such as tuberculosis can cause hypopituitarism. Neurosarcoidosis typically presents with DI. Systemic diseases can also cause functional hypopituitarism, but the significance of the disruption of pituitary function in this context is not always completely understood. Functional hypopituitarism in some cases is thought to be an appropriate response of the organism to insults. It is important to understand that some hormonal changes seen in admitted patients do not require treatment. One example frequently seen in the hospital is euthyroid sick syndrome, in which critically ill patients have functional secondary hypothyroidism with low TSH, T4, and T3 levels. Based on current knowledge, there is no indication for thyroid hormone replacement in these patients, and the thyroid hormone levels normalize when they recover from the acute phase of their illness. Chronically ill and malnourished patients frequently have central hypogonadism that also does not require treatment in the acute setting. For these reasons, it is not useful to measure gonadal and thyroid function in acutely ill patients. Similarly, the growth hormone axis is not assessed in hospitalized patients.

Genetic Causes

Mutations in several genes involved in pituitary development and differentiation, and hormone production and secretion are associated with isolated or combined pituitary hormone deficiency. Genetic defects in genes associated with pituitary gland development can also cause pituitary hypoplasia, aplasia, or other midline defects. Most of these patients have a known diagnosis of hypopituitarism upon admission to the hospital.

Vascular

Vascular events, including pituitary apoplexy and Sheehan's syndrome as discussed elsewhere, can also disrupt pituitary function.

Diagnosis of Hypopituitarism in the Hospital

The clinical manifestations of hypopituitarism can vary greatly depending on the axis affected, age, gender, and clinical status of the patient. Symptoms of hypopituitarism in acutely ill patients can be particularly challenging to recognize, given the masking of some subtle symptoms by other complications.

Assess Anterior Pituitary Function

Adrenal Axis

As stated above, central adrenal insufficiency must not be missed in a hospitalized patient given the risk that it poses to the patient's life. Patients with adrenal insufficiency may have longstanding nonspecific symptoms. In comparison with primary adrenal insufficiency, patients with central adrenal insufficiency have relative sparing of aldosterone secretion due to the preservation of renin and angiotensin control of aldosterone production. With this residual aldosterone production, severe hypotension and hyperkalemia are less common. Nonetheless, they can still present with hemodynamic instability despite adequate fluid resuscitation, most often associated with a hyperdynamic circulation and decreased systemic vascular resistance. This is an important diagnostic clue and should trigger investigation for adrenal insufficiency.

The combined occurrence of hypoglycemia, hyponatremia, and eosinophilia should alert the clinician to the possibility of hypoadrenalism. Patients with central adrenal insufficiency do not have the characteristic hyperpigmentation that classically occurs in patients with primary adrenal insufficiency, resulting from accumulation of proopiomelanocortin (POMC).

The diagnosis of adrenal insufficiency in the hospitalized patients is challenging not only because of the lack of specific symptoms or clinical signs but also due to the difficulties establishing cutoff values for cortisol levels in acutely ill patients. Expected cortisol levels vary with the type and severity of disease, making it difficult to define normal ranges. Patients admitted to the hospital do not have the classical circadian rhythms with higher cortisol levels early in the morning and lower levels at night. Many threshold levels have been proposed for the definition of an insufficient cortisol level (measured at any time of day) during acute illness, but none is entirely satisfactory. In critically ill patients, cortisol levels are usually elevated, and a serum cortisol value of ≥ 18 mcg/dL (497 nmol/L) effectively rules out adrenal insufficiency. Patients with central adrenal insufficiency have low cortisol levels with inappropriately normal or low ACTH levels. Given the lack of a cutoff value for random cortisol levels, an ACTH stimulation test can be performed to confirm the diagnosis of adrenal insufficiency if basal levels are equivocal. Cosyntropin, a synthetic ACTH corresponding to amino acids 1–24 of ACTH that has full biologic potency, is used to evaluate the capacity of the adrenal gland to produce cortisol. The ACTH stimulation or cosyntropin test consists of measuring serum cortisol immediately before and 30 and 60 minutes after intravenous or intramuscular injection of 250 mcg (85 nmol or 40 international units) of cosyntropin. Serum cortisol concentration ≥ 18 to 20 mcg/dL (500 to 550 nmol/L) after the injection indicates normal adrenal function. It is important to highlight that patients with new onset of central adrenal insufficiency may have an appropriate response to cosyntropin stimulation because the adrenal gland will respond to an ACTH stimulus normally. Therefore, a normal response to cosyntropin test does not rule out central adrenal insufficiency, and physicians will have to rely on basal cortisol and ACTH levels and clinical judgment. Patients with adrenal atrophy resulting from chronically low stimulation by endogenous ACTH will have an abnormal response in the cosyntropin test.

It is also important to note that hydrocortisone, prednisone, and several other corticosteroids cross-react with the assays used to measure cortisol and interfere with the assay results. Dexamethasone is not measured by the cortisol assays, but it is a strong inhibitor of the hypothalamic-pituitary axis and has a biological effect for almost 54 hours. For these reasons, cortisol levels should be interpreted with caution in patients who are currently receiving or recently received corticosteroids.

Thyroid Axis

As discussed above, the diagnosis of central hypothyroidism is challenging in the hospital, but thyroid hormone should be replaced in patients with secondary hypothyroidism in the hospital. If there is a clinical suspicion of pituitary dysfunction, TSH and FT4 should be measured. Patients with central hypothyroidism have low FT4 levels combined with inappropriately normal TSH levels. While this scenario can be seen in patients with "sick euthyroid syndrome," the presence of any known cause of hypopituitarism (see Table 2.1) would corroborate the diagnosis of central hypothyroidism.

Other Axes

Growth hormone and gonadotropin deficiencies usually do not pose risk to the patient's life, and thus there is usually no indication for testing these axes in hospitalized patients. Prolactin measurement can help diagnosing hypophysitis, as the levels can be low in this condition. All individuals with mechanical compression of the pituitary stalk can present with elevated prolactin levels; however, levels above 100 ng/dL are more suggestive of a prolactinoma. It is also important to keep in mind that several medications can increase prolactin levels.

Assess Posterior Pituitary Function

Patients with central DI are unable to concentrate urine. The diagnosis is particularly challenging in the hospital when patients frequently receive significant amounts of intravenous fluids for resuscitation and have increased volumes of dilute urine when fluid is being redistributed. True hypernatremia (plasma sodium concentration greater than 150 meq/L) is rare in adults with DI and no cognitive impairment, because the initial loss of water stimulates thirst, resulting in an increase in fluid intake to match the urinary losses. However, debilitated patients may not have free access to water, and some patients may have impaired thirst mechanisms. In this setting, the plasma sodium concentration can be elevated. Elevated serum sodium associated with low urine osmolality, particularly when urine osmolality is less than the plasma osmolality, is indicative of DI. The response to DDAVP treatment will differentiate between central and nephrogenic DI.

Imaging

Unless the patient has an unequivocal cause for a specific hormonal deficiency, patients should have imaging of the hypothalamic-pituitary region. Pituitary adenomas do not usually cause diabetes insipidus; this is usually caused by suprasellar lesions. Pituitary microadenomas do not usually cause hypopituitarism. Empty sella is a radiological term. It can be seen in association with pituitary hypoplasia/aplasia or can be a consequence of a previous insult to the pituitary gland such as apoplexy or hypophysitis. However, it can also be seen in patients with normal pituitary function. Absence of the posterior white spot may have no clinical significance or may be secondary to absence of ADH storage in the posterior hypophysis in patients with diabetes insipidus. Hypophysitis can present as enlargement of the pituitary gland and thickening of the stalk. However, normal imaging of the pituitary does not rule out hypophysitis.

Management of Hypopituitarism in the Hospital

Patients with a known diagnosis of hypopituitarism should continue their hormone replacement when admitted to the hospital, but some adjustments to the therapy are frequently necessary.

The most important treatment is corticosteroid therapy. Critically ill patients should receive stress dose steroids. A bolus of 100 mg of hydrocortisone followed by 50–100 mg IV every 6–8 hours is given; alternatively, 2–4 mg/h by continuous administration should be given. Dose should be tapered down to maintenance oral dose as the clinical condition improves.

Patients undergoing surgical procedures or immobilized patients at higher risk of deep venous thrombosis should discontinue estrogen therapy. Growth hormone and testosterone therapy are often discontinued during hospitalization, depending on specific situations. Thyroid replacement should be given to patients in the hospital, and special attention should be given to patients on enteral diets, given the need for it to be taken on an empty stomach for proper absorption. Patients with significant edema may have impaired absorption, and patients with proteinuria have increased wasting of thyroid hormones and may need adjustments in their dose of levothyroxine. Patients on DDVAP treatment should receive it while in the hospital and should be carefully monitored. Mental status alterations due to anesthesia or current disease can affect the thirst mechanism and interfere with appropriate water intake, requiring adjustment of the DDAVP dose. Patients are often NPO or have nasal tubes, and the DDAVP route of administration may need to be adjusted. If DDAVP cannot be administered intranasally or orally, it can be given subcutaneously or intravenously. A usual antidiuretic dose is 0.5 to 2 mcg administered subcutaneously or intravenously; the duration of action, as judged by increased urine osmolality, will be 12 hours or more. Some patients do not respond well to subcutaneous DDAVP due to inadequate absorption.

Management of Hypopituitarism at the Time of Discharge

Patients with hypopituitarism should be discharged on hormone replacement therapy. Patients on stress doses of steroids should be tapered to a replacement dose (around 3–4 mg of prednisone or 15 mg of hydrocortisone daily) as soon as they are clinically stable. Those with a new diagnosis of hormone deficiency should be reevaluated for the need of replacement therapy. If the diagnosis of hypopituitarism was made in an acute setting, after brain trauma or surgery, for example, patients may recover pituitary function and may not need long-term replacement or may need adjustment of dose of hormonal replacement. The appropriate time for post-discharge follow-up will depend on the specific hormonal deficiency and the cause of hypopituitarism. A follow-up visit 6 weeks after discharge to evaluate pituitary status may be ideal in most cases.

Suggested Reading

Benvenga S, Campenni A, Ruggeri RM, Trimarchi F. Clinical review 113: Hypopituitarism secondary to head trauma. J Clin Endocrinol Metabol. 2000;85:1353–61.

Caturegli P, Newschaffer C, Olivi A, Pomper MG, Burger PC, Rose NR. Autoimmune hypophysitis. Endocr Rev. 2005;26:599–614.

Schneider HJ, Aimaretti G, Kreitschmann-Andermahr I, Stalla GK, Ghigo E. Hypopituitarism. Lancet. 2007;369:1461–70.

Thodou E, Asa SL, Kontogeorgos G, Kovacs K, Horvath E, Ezzat S. Clinical case seminar: lymphocytic hypophysitis: clinicopathological findings. J Clin Endocrinol Metabol. 1995;80:2302–11.

Postoperative Management After Pituitary Surgery

3

Anna Zelfond Feldman
and Pamela Hartzband

Contents

A. Z. Feldman (✉)
Harvard Medical School, Beth Israel Deaconess Medical Center,
Department of Endocrinology, Boston, MA, USA
e-mail: afeldma1@bidmc.harvard.edu

P. Hartzband
Harvard Medical School, Beth Israel Deaconess Medical Center,
Department of Endocrinology and Metabolism, Boston, MA, USA
e-mail: phartzba@bidmc.harvard.edu

© Springer Nature Switzerland AG 2020
R. K. Garg et al. (eds.), *Handbook of Inpatient Endocrinology*,
https://doi.org/10.1007/978-3-030-38976-5_3

Assess Hormone Status Before Surgery if Possible

– Ideally patient should be seen by endocrinology as outpatient prior to surgery.

Intraoperative/Postoperative Steroids

Patient with *Unknown Adrenal Function* Prior to Surgery

– **Day of surgery (pre- or intra-op):** Hydrocortisone 100 mg IV q 8 h (alternative methylprednisolone 60 mg IV × 1).
– **POD 1:** Hydrocortisone 100 mg IV × 1 at 8 am and hydrocortisone 50 mg IV × 1 at 4 pm (alternative methylprednisolone 30 mg IV × 1), and then hold steroids.
– **POD 2:** Draw 8 am fasting cortisol level. After blood is drawn (while results pending), give hydrocortisone 50 mg IV q 12 h (alternative methylprednisolone 20 mg IV × 1).
– **POD 3:** If a.m. cortisol drawn on POD 2 is >/= 10, stop steroids.

  If a.m. cortisol drawn on POD 2 is <10 (or results pending, or patient received steroids within 12 hours prior to cortisol assessment), start oral hydrocortisone 15 mg morning and 5 mg afternoon (alternative prednisone 5 mg morning). Higher doses of steroids may be needed depending on clinical status.
– **Discharge:** Discharge patient on hydrocortisone or prednisone if indicated as above.
– Additional outpatient assessment of HPA axis should be done in approximately 2 weeks at endocrine follow-up.

Patients Known to Have *Preexisting Adrenal Insufficiency*

- **Day of surgery (pre-op):** hydrocortisone 100 mg IV q 8 h (alternative methylprednisolone 60 mg IV × 1).
- **POD 1:** Hydrocortisone 50 mg IV × q 8 h (alternative methyl-prednisolone 30 mg IV × 1).
- **POD 2:** Hydrocortisone 50 mg IV q 12 h (alternative methyl-prednisolone 20 mg IV × 1).
- **POD 3:** Start oral hydrocortisone 15 mg morning and 5 mg afternoon (alternative prednisone 5 mg morning). Higher doses of steroids may be needed depending on clinical status.
- **Discharge:** No assessment of adrenal function in the hospital; patient should be discharged on steroids as above.

Patients Known to Have *Normal Adrenal Function Preoperatively* and Patients with *Cushing's Disease*

- **Day of surgery:** Do not give pre-, peri-, or postoperative glucocorticoids.
- Monitor patient closely for adrenal insufficiency.
- **POD 1:** Check 8 a.m. fasting cortisol. After blood is drawn (while results pending), give hydrocortisone 50 mg IV × q 8 h (alternative methylprednisolone 30 mg IV × 1).
- **POD 2**: If a.m. cortisol drawn on POD 2 is >/= 10, stop steroids.

  If a.m. cortisol drawn on POD 2 is <10 (or results pending or patient received steroids within 12 hours prior to cortisol assessment), give hydrocortisone 50 mg IV q 12 hours (alternative methylprednisolone 20 mg IV × 1).

- **POD 3: If patient still on steroids:** Start oral hydrocortisone 15 mg morning and 5 mg afternoon (alternative prednisone 5 mg morning). Higher doses of steroids may be needed depending on clinical status.
- **Discharge:** Endocrinologist to follow up 8 a.m. cortisol drawn on POD1 prior to discharge and decide on steroid management.

Diabetes Insipidus/Sodium Management

- **Day of surgery**: Check serum Na and urine osmolality or specific gravity post-op.
- **POD 1–2**: Check serum Na and urine osmolality or specific gravity bid. Increase frequency if clinically indicated. Reduce to daily if clinically stable.
  - **Strict ins/outs** with special attention to **urine output (UOP)**: Urine output should be measured hourly (if catheter) or Q 2 hours (if no catheter) postoperatively.
  - If **UOP is >250 cc/h × 2 or more hours**: Send serum Na and urine osmolality or specific gravity.
- If labs consistent with DI with **Na >145 with urine specific gravity <1.005 or osmolality <300**:
  - Give DDAVP 1 mcg IV × 1.
  - If patient getting NS IVF, change IVF to one-half NS (alternative D5W).
  - Monitor serum Na, urine osmolality, or specific gravity q 4–6 hours until either DI resolves or Na normalizes and is stable, and then decrease frequency of labs.
  - Repeated doses of DDAVP IV may be needed. However, DI post-transsphenoidal surgery is often transient. If DI is persistent, patient may need oral daily, BID, or rarely TID doses of DDAVP. Intranasal DDAVP is contraindicated in the immediate postoperative period.

- If discordant labs with **Na >145 with urine specific gravity >1.005 or osmolality >300** or **Na normal with urine specific gravity <1.005 or osmolality <300:**
  - Monitor closely, but DDAVP is not necessarily indicated.
  - Clinical judgment must be used in these cases about DDAVP administration.
- **Discontinue IVF** as quickly as possible and allow patient to drink to thirst.
  - If thirst mechanism is not intact, match PO intake to urine output.
- **Discharge**: If DI is persistent and patient is discharged on oral DDAVP, a serum Na level should be checked within 1–2 days of discharge, as some patients will develop transient syndrome of inappropriate diuretic hormone secretion (SIADH).
  - These patients need close follow-up postoperatively, ideally within 1 week of discharge.

Arrange Endocrine Follow-Up Within 1–2 Weeks of Discharge

- Order **8 a.m. cortisol and Na** to be done fasting 1–2 days prior to endocrine follow-up.
  - If the patient is *discharged on hydrocortisone*, advise patient to hold this medication the afternoon prior and the morning of the lab draw and to take it immediately after labs are drawn that morning.
  - If the patient is *discharged on prednisone*, advise patient to hold this medication on day of lab draw and take it immediately after labs are drawn that morning.
- Urine osmolality or specific gravity may also be ordered if clinically indicated.

Suggested Reading

Fleseriu M, Hashim IA, Karavitaki N, Melmed S, Murad MH, Salvatori R, Samuels MH. Hormonal replacement in hypopituitarism in adults: an endocrine society clinical practice guideline. J Clin Endocrinol Metabol. 2016;101(11):3888–921.

Woodmansee WW, Carmichael J, Kelly D, Katznelson L. AACE Neuroendocrine and Pituitary Scientific Committee. American Association of Clinical Endocrinologists and American College of Endocrinology Disease State Clinical Review: Postoperative Management Following Pituitary Surgery. Endocr Pract. 2015;21(7):832–8.

Ziu M, Dunn IF, Hess C, Fleseriu M, Bodach ME, Tumialan LM, et al. Congress of neurological surgeons systematic review and evidence-based guideline on posttreatment follow-up evaluation of patients with nonfunctioning pituitary adenomas. Neurosurgery. 2016;79(4):E541–3.

Severe Thyrotoxicosis and Thyroid Storm

4

Melissa G. Lechner and Trevor E. Angell

Contents

M. G. Lechner
David Geffen School of Medicine, University of California at Los
Angeles, Division of Endocrinology, Diabetes and Metabolism,
Los Angeles, CA, USA
e-mail: mlechner@mednet.ucla.edu

T. E. Angell (✉)
Keck School of Medicine, University of Southern California, Division of
Endocrinology and Diabetes, Los Angeles, CA, USA
e-mail: trevor.angell@med.usc.edu

© Springer Nature Switzerland AG 2020
R. K. Garg et al. (eds.), *Handbook of Inpatient Endocrinology*,
https://doi.org/10.1007/978-3-030-38976-5_4

Performing the History for Thyrotoxicosis

Assess Symptoms of Thyrotoxicosis

Symptoms of thyrotoxicosis frequently include sweating, heat
intolerance, palpitations, fatigue, and dyspnea on exertion.
Cognitive symptoms may include anxiety, hyperactivity, or diffi-
culty with concentration. Reported weight loss may be modest or
substantial. Note any previous history of Graves' disease, other
thyroid disorders, thyroid surgery, and radioactive iodine treatment. In *apathetic hyperthyroidism*, overt symptoms are absent or
often limited to weight loss, failure to thrive, fatigue, or lethargy.
In patients already taking β-blockers, thyrotoxic symptoms may
be blunted.

Assess for the Etiology of Thyrotoxicosis

Patients with longer duration of symptoms (>3 months) likely
have persistent hyperthyroidism such as Graves' disease or autonomous nodule(s). Patients may report diffuse thyroid enlargement

in Graves' disease, a tender thyroid in subacute (painful) thyroiditis, or a history of thyroid nodules suggesting possible autonomous function. Eye complaints (protrusion, inflammation, or visual changes) are seen only in Graves' disease.

Assess for Medications That Affect Thyroid Status

Note use of thyroid hormone preparations, antithyroid medication (methimazole or propylthiouracil [PTU]), exposure to iodinated contrast or iodine supplements, weight loss supplements, or other medications, including amiodarone, lithium, tyrosine kinase inhibitors, and immune checkpoint inhibitors for cancer treatment.

Performing the Physical Exam for Thyrotoxicosis

Key Findings in Thyrotoxicosis

Findings include sweating, skin warmth, fine tremor, low body weight and loss of muscle mass, hyperactivity, and poor attention. Heart rate (HR) may be mildly elevated (80–100 bpm) or clearly tachycardic. Supraventricular tachyarrhythmias, particularly atrial fibrillation, or signs of heart failure may be present. There is often mild systolic hypertension with widened pulse pressure. Patients may be mildly tachypneic from thyrotoxicosis alone. Rarely, patients may present with episodes of paralysis (termed *paroxysmal periodic paralysis*), affecting the lower before the upper extremities, proximal more than distal muscle groups, and usually sparing the diaphragm.

Specific Exam Findings in Different Causes of Thyrotoxicosis

A diffusely enlarged non-tender thyroid gland suggests Graves' disease, and the presence of a thyroid bruit in combination with ophthalmopathy, pretibial myxedema, or digital clubbing is pathognomonic. Exquisite thyroid tenderness indicates subacute (painful) thyroiditis. The presence of a large thyroid nodule on palpation may suggest an autonomously functioning nodule. The presence of a normal or small thyroid gland without any abnormal characteristics in the appropriate clinical setting may suggest accidental or surreptitious patient use of thyroid hormones.

Assessing for Thyroid Storm

The critical physical exam findings include hyperthermia, altered mentation (e.g., confusion, lethargy, seizures, coma), tachyarrhythmias (most commonly atrial fibrillation), or congestive heart failure (e.g., elevated jugular venous pressure, lower extremity swelling, pulmonary edema, congestive hepatopathy). Other features of thyrotoxicosis described above will often be present in patients with thyroid storm but are not specific and frequently present in thyrotoxic patients without thyroid storm as well.

Making a Diagnosis of Thyroid Storm

Thyroid storm is a clinical diagnosis. Thyroid storm has been recognized traditionally as a clinical syndrome of thyrotoxicosis, hyperthermia, altered mentation, and a precipitating event. Other manifestations of thyrotoxicosis are often present but are not specific for thyroid storm. The **Burch-Wartofsky Score** assigns points for dysfunction of the thermoregulatory, central nervous, gastrointestinal (GI)-hepatic, and cardiovascular systems. A score of >45 is considered highly suspicious for thyroid storm. However, this cutoff is not specific, indicating that some thyrotoxic patients without thyroid storm have a score greater than 45. The numerical score should not supplant physician judgment in making the diagnosis.

Obtain Thyroid Function Tests

Biochemical assessments of thyroid function are the most pertinent laboratory results to consider. A suppressed thyroid-stimulating hormone (**TSH**) helps establish thyrotoxicosis. Thyroid hormone measurement, such as free thyroxine (**FT4**), should also be performed to confirm thyroid hormone excess, since mild TSH suppression in hospitalized patients occurs with non-thyroidal illnesses. Biochemical confirmation of thyrotoxicosis is not necessary to diagnose and begin treatment for thyroid storm. The degree of thyroid hormone elevation or other tests are not helpful in determining which thyrotoxic patients have thyroid storm.

Biochemical Findings in Thyrotoxicosis

Mild hyperglycemia, hypercalcemia, normocytic anemia, and elevation in alkaline phosphatase and transaminase concentrations are all commonly seen in thyrotoxicosis. Serum creatinine is lower in thyrotoxicosis, leading to overestimating glomerular filtrate rate. An elevated bilirubin is a particularly important finding since it has been correlated with adverse outcomes in thyroid storm.

Obtain Testing to Identify Underlying Illnesses

It is most critical to identify concurrent illnesses that may complicate thyrotoxicosis or be precipitants of thyroid storm. In addition to a thorough physical exam, pregnancy test should be performed if relevant, and sources of infection should be assessed through urinalysis, blood cultures, and chest imaging. Consideration of concomitant adrenal insufficiency should be assessed with a random serum cortisol, but doing so should not delay delivery of steroid treatment (discussed below). If adrenal insufficiency is suspected, more formal evaluation, such as a cosyntropin (ACTH 1–24) stimulation test, may need to be deferred until recovery from the patient's acute presentation. Further testing, such as abdominal imaging or lumbar puncture, should be performed when clinically indicated. Other testing should evaluate for potential acute coronary syndrome, hyperglycemia and diabetic keto-acidosis, and drug use (especially cocaine and methamphetamines).

Initial Emergent Therapy for Thyroid Storm or Severe Thyrotoxicosis

The treatment of thyroid storm should be initiated as early as possible after recognition of the diagnosis. For patients with severe thyrotoxicosis who are considered to have "impending" thyroid storm based on clinical evaluation or a BWS of 25–45, similar treatment to thyroid storm may be considered.

Provide Aggressive Supportive Care

- Hemodynamic stabilization is critical. Management in the intensive care unit (ICU) is usually needed for patients with thyroid storm. Invasive hemodynamic monitoring is often appropriate. Intravenous fluid is typically necessary to improve perfusion in the setting of absolute or effective hypovolemia. If hypotension is not responsive to fluid resuscitation, vasopressors should be used.
- Sedatives, narcotics, and diuretics should be used carefully because they may lower blood pressure and worsen hypoperfusion.
- Hyperthermia can initially be treated with cooling measures and acetaminophen. Salicylates may increase free hormone levels by lowering protein binding.

- Underlying illnesses should be treated. Specifically, broad-spectrum empiric antibiotics should be considered given the frequency with which infections precipitate thyroid storm.

Order β-Blocker Therapy

β-Adrenergic blockade improves tachycardia, cardiac workload, oxygen demand, and thyrotoxic symptoms. The HR goal is approximately 90–110 bpm rather than slower rates until thyrotoxicosis resolves. Carefully monitoring and use of shorter-acting agents may reduce the risk of cardiovascular insufficiency arising from excess β-blockade.

Initial regimens include the following:

- Intravenous **propranolol** 0.5–1.0 mg and then continuous infusion (5–10 mg/hour)
- Oral **propranolol** 60–80 mg every 4 hours
- Intravenous esmolol 0.25–0.50 mg/kg loading dose and then continuous infusion (0.05–0.1 mg/kg/minute)

Order Antithyroid Drug Therapy

Start antithyroid drugs at least *1 hour before* iodides to prevent iodine incorporation into additional thyroid hormone. Initial regimens include the following:

- PTU (oral loading dose of 500–1000 mg and then 250 mg every 4 hours) is favored for thyroid storm, because it decreases peripheral conversion of T4 to T3.
- Methimazole (oral 60–80 mg daily) is an alternative when there is endogenous hyperthyroidism (e.g., Graves' disease), but does not inhibit peripheral convention.

- When a patient is unable to take medication orally, nasogastric tube (NGT) administration may be employed. If there are contraindications to NGT use or other issues that limit upper GI function, an intravenous reconstitution of methimazole in 0.9% saline solution given as a slow IV push has been reported. Per rectum regimens also have been employed (see also Chap. 7).

Order Iodine Therapy

Because thyroidal exposure to excess iodine acutely attenuates thyroid hormone secretion, consideration should be given to initiating an inorganic iodine preparation, such as saturated solution of potassium iodide [**SSKI**] (250 mg [0.25 ml/drop] every 6 hours). Iodines produce rapid decrease in thyroidal hormone release and can lower circulating thyroid hormone levels to near normal within 4–5 days. Again, to prevent incorporation of iodine in newly formed thyroid hormone and potentially prolong or exacerbate hyperthyroidism, antithyroid medication should be given *before* initiation of iodine therapy (see above).

Order Steroid Therapy

Give glucocorticoid therapy (intravenous **hydrocortisone** 300 mg and then 100 mg every 8 hours) to reduce T4 to T3 conversion and potentially treat coexisting adrenal insufficiency.

Use of Adjunct Treatments in Refractory Cases

Other treatments have been used in cases where patients are unable to receive traditional treatment or remain critically ill despite therapy. The data supporting these measures are limited.

- **Calcium channel blockers.** Verapamil and diltiazem, which are not dihydropyridines and therefore do not cause vasodilator-induced reflex tachycardia, have been used for rate control in lieu of, but not in combination with, β-blockers.

- **Cholestyramine.** When used with thionamides and a β-blocker, serum T4 and T3 levels drop faster during the first 2 weeks of therapy.
- **Lithium** carbonate (300 mg every 6 hours and titration to lithium level of 0.8–1.2 mEq/L) causes inhibition of thyroid hormone release from the thyroid.
- **Plasmapheresis** (2.5– 3 L volume of combined fresh-frozen plasma and 5% albumin) can remove excess thyroid hormone from circulation.
- **L-carnitine** (1–2 g twice daily) may inhibit T3 action in the nucleus.
- **Thyroidectomy** may be necessary in rare patients to treat hyperthyroidism when medical therapy does not adequately control thyrotoxicosis.

Treatment of Thyrotoxic Patients Without Thyroid Storm

- Hospitalized thyrotoxic patients usually require prompt but not emergent therapy. Providing β-blockers, such as propranolol (orally 10–40 mg every 8 hours), ameliorates adrenergic symptoms. Initial dosing should be based on blood pressure and heart rate tolerability and the presence of CHF. Initiation of methimazole for patients diagnosed with Graves' disease during hospitalization may be appropriate.

Monitoring Clinical Response

After initiation of therapy, supportive care measures should be adjusted to treat hemodynamic status as needed. Titration of β-blocker therapy should be performed to goal heart rates while avoiding hypotension. Repeat assessment of circulating thyroid hormone levels may be helpful to assure improvement starting 2–3 days after treatment initiation.

Planning Outpatient Follow-Up

Discharge plans should include a timely follow-up visit with an endocrinologist for continued treatment. In Graves' disease, interruption of therapy can result in recurrence of symptoms. Patients should be advised about common adverse effects, which are most often rash, itching, GI upset, taste change, and joint pain. Agranulocytosis, vasculitis, hepatic inflammation, and cholestasis are rare but potentially life-threatening complications of antithyroid drugs, and patients should be informed to report relevant symptoms. Repeat thyroid hormone testing should be performed 2–4 weeks after discharge to assure improvement in thyrotoxicosis. Once stable, definitive treatment (radioactive iodine ablation or thyroidectomy) may be warranted for patients with Graves' disease to prevent recurrent hospitalization for thyrotoxicosis.

Disclosure Statement All authors have no financial disclosures.

Suggested Reading

Alfadhli E, Gianoukakis AG. Management of severe thyrotoxicosis when the gastrointestinal tract is compromised. Thyroid. 2011;21(3):215–20.

Angell TE, Lechner MG, Nguyen CT, Salvato VL, Nicoloff JT, LoPresti JS. Clinical features and hospital outcomes in thyroid storm: a retrospective cohort study. J Clin Endocrinol Metab. 2015;100(2):451–9.

Burch HB, Wartofsky L. Life-threatening thyrotoxicosis. Thyroid storm. Endocrinol Metab Clin North Am. 1993;22(2):263–77.

Klein I, Danzi S. Thyroid disease and the heart. Curr Probl Cardiol. 2016;41(2):65–92.

Klubo-Gwiezdzinska J, Wartofsky L. Thyroid emergencies. Med Clin North Am. 2012;96(2):385–403.

Ross DS, Burch HB, Cooper DS, Greenlee MC, Laurberg P, Maia AL, Rivkees SA, Samuels M, Sosa JA, Stan MN, Walter MA. American thyroid association guidelines for diagnosis and management of hyperthyroidism and other causes of thyrotoxicosis. Thyroid. 2016;26(10):1343–421.

Myxedema Coma

5

Gwendolyne Anyanate Jack and James V. Hennessey

Contents

G. A. Jack (✉)
Weill Cornell Medical Center-New York Presbyterian Hospital,
Department of Medicine, Division of Endocrinology, Diabetes and
Metabolism, New York, NY, USA
e-mail: gwj9003@med.cornell.edu

J. V. Hennessey
Beth Israel Deaconess Medical Center, Harvard Medical School,
Division of Endocrinology, Diabetes and Metabolism,
Boston, MA, USA
e-mail: jhenness@bidmc.harvard.edu

© Springer Nature Switzerland AG 2020
R. K. Garg et al. (eds.), *Handbook of Inpatient Endocrinology*,
https://doi.org/10.1007/978-3-030-38976-5_5

Abbreviations

AST	aspartate aminotransferase
ATA	American Thyroid Association
GCS	Glasgow Coma Scale
GFR	glomerular filtration rate
LDH	Lactate dehydrogenase
LDL	Low-density lipoprotein
LT3	Liothyronine
LT4	Levothyroxine
MC	Myxedema coma
NTI	Nonthyroidal illness
T3	Triiodothyronine
T4	Thyroxine
TSH	Thyroid-stimulating hormone

Assess Preadmission Thyroid Status and Thyroid Treatment

Since patients present with altered mentation, obtaining a history may be difficult. Therefore, it is also important to obtain collateral information from family, friends, and outpatient medical records.

A detailed history may reveal underlying hypothyroidism, previous history of thyroidectomy (with thyroidectomy scar on exam), radioactive iodine ablation (RAI), and medication noncompliance/inappropriate discontinuation of thyroid hormone therapy. Signs and symptoms such as lapses in memory, slowness of thoughts, disorientation, fatigue, cold intolerance, weight gain, edema, constipation, brittle nails, and thin/coarse hair may be present. Vital signs may show hypothermia, hypotension, and bradycardia. Some patients may have undiagnosed hypothyroidism; therefore, other physical exam findings typical of hypothyroidism may provide clues such as the presence of a goiter, cold dry skin, delayed reflex relaxation phase, periorbital edema, facial puffiness, non-pitting edema in the upper and lower extremities, and enlarged tongue.

Evaluate for Risk Factors Associated with Myxedema Coma

In addition to determining if the patient has not been taking thyroid hormone or taking it improperly, it is important to evaluate for other precipitating factors such as infection, cold exposure, heart failure, myocardial infarction, cerebrovascular accident, trauma, surgery, gastrointestinal bleed, substantial iodine intake such as from chronic raw bok choy consumption, and several culprit medications such as amiodarone, lithium, phenytoin, sedatives, antidepressants, and anesthetics.

Identify Cardinal Features of Myxedema Coma

Myxedema coma should be suspected in a patient with decreased mental status, hypothermia (which can be as low as core temperature < 80 °F), and bradycardia, in addition to clinical signs/symptoms of hypothyroidism, especially in older women during the winter months.

Use a Systems-Based Approach to Identify Multi-organ Dysfunction

General

As discussed, hypothermia is one of the key features of myxedema coma. It is important to note that in the setting of underlying infection, patients may be normothermic due to blunted ability to mount a febrile response in the setting of thermal dysregulation. Typical signs of infection (fever, tachycardia, diaphoresis) may not be evident. Therefore in a patient with suspected myxedema coma, normal temperature should warrant more in-depth investigation for underlying infection. Complete blood count with differential, urinalysis, urine culture, and blood culture should be obtained (Table 5.1).

Neurologic

Neurocognitive disturbances observed in myxedema include a reduced level of consciousness, confusion, psychomotor slowing, cerebellar ataxia, memory deficits, dementia, depression, seizure, lethargy that devolves into stupor, and ultimately coma. Sensory and motor peripheral neuropathy, psychosis, and hallucinations ("myxedema madness") have also been described.

Cardiovascular

Cardiovascular disturbances include reduction in myocardial contractility, low cardiac output, hypotension, cardiogenic shock, and bradycardia. Mucopolysaccharide accumulation in the pericardium can lead to pericardial effusions and subsequent cardiac tamponade physiology. Patients may endorse dyspnea. Physical exam would reveal jugular venous distention, muffled heart sounds, tachycardia, and pulsus paradoxus and can be further confirmed by chest X-ray, EKG, and cardiac echocardiogram. Confirmatory tests include chest X-ray, EKG, and cardiac echocardiogram.

Table 5.1 Signs and symptoms of myxedema coma

	Signs/symptoms
General	Fatigue, weakness
	Hypothermia without shivering
Neurologic	Memory deficits
	Delayed relaxation phase of DTR
	Seizure
	Psychomotor slowing
	Decreased level of consciousness (lethargy, stupor, coma)
Cardiac	Bradycardia (tachycardia if cardiac tamponade is present)
	Hypotension
	Diastolic dysfunction
	Tamponade
Respiratory	Dyspnea
Renal	Decreased urine output
	Bladder atony
	Increased creatinine
	Decreased GFR
Metabolic	Hypoglycemia
	Hyponatremia
	Elevated creatine kinase, elevated LDH
	Elevated LDL
Gastrointestinal	Constipation, fecal impaction
	Paralytic ileus, megacolon
	Ascites
	Elevated AST
Dermatologic	Puffy face and extremities
	Cool, dry skin
	Cold intolerance
	Brittle nails
	Thin, sparse, dry hair
Musculoskeletal	Myalgia, easy fatigability

Respiratory

Respiratory manifestations including hypoventilation, hypoxia, and hypercapnia can also occur in myxedema coma patients. An arterial blood gas analysis to assess for hypercapnia and hypoxemia should be considered. Also, laryngeal edema and macroglossia, resulting in airway narrowing, can pose a challenge during endotracheal tube placement. Pleural effusions and underlying pneumonia can also contribute to diminished respiratory function. Chest X-ray should be obtained to evaluate for underlying pneumonia and pleural effusion.

Gastrointestinal

Bowel wall edema can result in reduced intestinal motility, atony, paralytic ileus, and toxic megacolon. Patients may present with nausea/vomiting, abdominal distension, constipation, and fecal impaction. Also, absorption of medications can be diminished, and dose adjustment of oral medications may be needed. Impaired gluconeogenesis, infection, and concomitant adrenal insufficiency may contribute to hypoglycemia; therefore, serum blood sugar should be obtained.

Genitourinary

Severe hypothyroidism results in a decrease in renal glomerular filtration rate and renal perfusion and rhabdomyolysis. Obtain a complete metabolic panel, which may reveal hyponatremia, elevated creatinine kinase, creatinine, and aspartate aminotransferase. Urine output should also be monitored for decreased urine output from acute renal injury and bladder atony.

Order Thyroid Function Tests. Do Not Wait for Results

The diagnosis of myxedema coma is in large part based on clinical suspicion and confirmed with biochemical testing. Thyroid function tests including thyroid-stimulating hormone (TSH), free T4 (fT4), should be obtained prior to administration of thyroid replacement therapy. Initial evaluation includes an assessment of underlying precipitating factors; however, if a high index of suspicion is obvious, do not wait until the results of the evaluation are definitive before initiating treatment.

Order Cortisol for Adrenal Insufficiency Evaluation. Do Not Wait for Results

Given the overlap in the presentation of MC with adrenal insufficiency such as fatigue, hyponatremia, hypothermia, and hypoglycemia, evaluation for adrenal insufficiency is prudent. Adrenal insufficiency can be from hypopituitarism or can be part of polyendocrine syndrome in a patient with underlying Hashimoto's thyroiditis with autoimmune primary adrenal insufficiency (i.e., Schmidt syndrome). Also, after starting thyroid replacement therapy, there is concern for increased metabolism of cortisol leading to adrenal crisis; therefore, obtaining baseline serum cortisol level is essential. In a stressed patient with normal serum albumin levels, a serum cortisol level greater than 18 mg/dl would rule out adrenal insufficiency and would permit rapid taper of hydrocortisone after limited initial exposure.

Admit Critically Ill Patients to Intensive Care Unit for Close Monitoring

Myxedema crisis is an emergency that warrants frequent monitoring of patient's clinical status; therefore, it should be managed in a critical care setting.

Provide Emergency Supportive Care

Maintain a low threshold for intubation and mechanical ventilation in the setting of worsening hypoxemia and hypercapnia and concern for airway protection in the setting of reduced Glasgow Coma Scale, macroglossia, or suspicion for laryngeal edema.

Cardiovascular collapse and hypotension may require volume resuscitation with isotonic normal saline or 5–10% dextrose in half-normal saline if hypoglycemia is also present. Hypotension might be refractory to intravenous fluids without thyroid replacement therapy and in the setting of adrenal insufficiency. Vasopressors may be added if fluid resuscitation is inadequate in providing cardiovascular support; however, it should be weaned off as soon as clinically indicated.

Regarding management of hypothermia, external warming techniques with blankets are suitable, though this may worsen hypotension through vasodilation. Aggressive external rewarming and central warming can potentiate cardiovascular collapse; therefore, it is generally not recommended. Treatment with thyroid hormone should restore thermoregulation.

Administer Stress Dose Glucocorticoids

Due to the concern for underlying adrenal insufficiency, and the risk of inciting adrenal crisis with initiation of thyroid hormone therapy, it is recommended that stress dose steroids be administered prior to thyroid supplementation. Hydrocortisone 50–100 mg can be administered intravenously every 6–8 hours until clinical improvement and quickly tapered off if labs obtained prior to glucocorticoid initiation ultimately do not demonstrate adrenal insufficiency.

Manage Underlying Precipitating Factors

Based on clinical presentation, laboratory analysis, and imaging studies, treat for any precipitants such as myocardial infarction, gastrointestinal bleeding, and other underlying medical conditions. If suspicious for infection, draw cultures and start empiric antibiotics. Metabolic derangements such as hypoglycemia and hyponatremia should be monitored and treated accordingly. Caution must be exercised to not rapidly correct serum sodium, given the risk for osmotic demyelination syndrome. This is focused on the classic definition; however, a similar approach can be adopted in patients with features of profound hypothyroidism.

Administer Levothyroxine +/− LT3

Controversy exists regarding optimal thyroid hormone regimens including the type, dose, route, frequency of administration, and duration of therapy. An approach adopted by earlier studies is administration of an intravenous L-thyroxine 300–600 µg loading dose to replete the deficit in the total body thyroid hormone pool, followed by maintenance doses of 50–100 µg LT4 daily by intravenous or oral route (if mentally alert). The ATA 2014 guideline recommends an intravenous loading dose *of 200–400 µg of L-thyroxine, followed by daily oral L-thyroxine dose of 1.6 µg/kg body weight or 75% of this dose if intravenous route.* The underlying principle behind levothyroxine monotherapy is that it allows for restoration to near-normal levels.

In myxedema coma, T3 is low and concomitant nonthyroidal illness further decreases T4 to T3 conversion. Therefore, another strategy is the addition of LT3 to L-thyroxine therapy. LT3 has a quicker onset on action, crosses the blood-brain barrier readily, increases core temperature within 2–3 hours (as opposed to 14 hours from LT4 intravenously), and possibly improves neuropsychiatric manifestations more rapidly. According to the ATA 2014 guidelines, clinicians can consider coadministration of LT3, with an initial intravenous loading dose of LT3 5–20 µg, followed by a maintenance dose of LT3 IV 2.5–10 µg every 8 hours, which can be continued until patient's clinical status has improved and maintenance oral LT4 can be administered. Alternatively, LT3 therapy can be added if clinical status does not improve after 24–48 hours of L-thyroxine alone. Due to the potential risk of cardiac arrhythmias and myocardial infarction, especially in older patients, it is recommended to use lower doses of L-thyroxine and LT3.

Follow Up the Results of Thyroid Function Tests and Cortisol

Marked TSH elevation is consistent with primary hypothyroidism. In patients with central hypothyroidism, TSH is not a reliable measure. Also, TSH may not be substantially elevated in the setting of nonthyroidal illness (NTI) and glucocorticoid or dopamine administration. In myxedema coma, free T4 is low, and with concomitant nonthyroidal illness, these parameters may be even lower. In those known to be hypothyroid or with well-established hypothyroidism, if thyroid function tests and cortisol are normal, glucocorticoids can be promptly discontinued, and depending on clinical status, one may consider transitioning to the preadmission LT4 dose.

Reassess Clinical Status of Patient

It is important to monitor the patient frequently for clinical improvement. Once stabilized, frequent monitoring is no longer necessary, and patient can be transferred to medical floors for further management.

Hospital Discharge Plan

Patients with underlying hypothyroidism should be instructed to administer levothyroxine on an empty stomach and wait at least 1 hour before eating/drinking, in order to optimize absorption of LT4. If dose adjustments of LT4 were done during hospitalization, repeat TSH can be obtained in 6–8 weeks to determine if further dosage adjustments are needed. Outpatient follow-up with the patient's endocrinologist and primary care physician should be arranged to reassess thyroid status at an appropriate interval.

Suggested Reading

Chiong YV, Bammerlin E, Mariash CN. Development of an objective tool for the diagnosis of myxedema coma. Transl Res. 2015;166(3):233–43.
Fliers E, Wiersinga WM. Myxedema coma. Rev Endocr Metab Disord. 2003;4(2):137–41.
Holvey DN, Goodner CJ, Nicoloff JT, Dowling JT. Treatment of myxedema coma with intravenous thyroxine. Arch Intern Med. 1964;113(1):89–96.
Jordan RM. Myxedema coma: pathophysiology, therapy, and factors affecting prognosis. Med Clin N Am. 1995;79(1):185–94.

Kasid N, Hennessey JV. Myxedema Coma. In: Endocrine and metabolic medical emergencies: a clinician's guide; 2018. p. 252–61.

Klubo-Gwiezdzinska J, Wartofsky L. Thyroid emergencies. Med Clin N Am. 2012;96(2):385–403.

Liamis G, Filippatos TD, Liontos A, Elisaf MS. Management of endocrine disease: Hypothyroidism-associated hyponatremia: mechanisms, implications and treatment. Eur J Endocrinol. 2017;176(1):R15–r20.

Mathew V, Misgar RA, Ghosh S, Mukhopadhyay P, Roychowdhury P, Pandit K, et al. Myxedema coma: a new look into an old crisis. J Thyroid Res. 2011;2011:493462.

Osborn LA, Skipper B, Arellano I, MacKerrow SD, Crawford MH. Results of resting and ambulatory electrocardiograms in patients with hypothyroidism and after return to euthyroid status. Heart Dis. 1999;1(1):8–11.

Popoveniuc G, Chandra T, Sud A, Sharma M, Blackman MR, Burman KD, et al. A diagnostic scoring system for myxedema coma. Endocr Pract. 2014;20(8):808–17.

Sorensen JR, Winther KH, Bonnema SJ, Godballe C, Hegedus L. Respiratory manifestations of hypothyroidism: a systematic review. Thyroid. 2016;26(11):1519–27.

Wartofsky L. Myxedema coma. Endocrinol Metab Clin N Am. 2006;35(4):687–98, vii-viii.

Abnormal Thyroid Stimulating Hormone Values That Are Not due to Common Causes of Primary Hypothyroidism or Thyrotoxicosis

6

Zsu-Zsu Chen and James V. Hennessey

Contents

Z.-Z. Chen (✉)
Beth Israel Deaconess Medical Center, Department of Endocrinology,
Diabetes and Metabolism, Boston, MA, USA
e-mail: zchen5@bidmc.harvard.edu

J. V. Hennessey
Beth Israel Deaconess Medical Center, Harvard Medical School,
Division of Endocrinology, Diabetes and Metabolism,
Boston, MA, USA
e-mail: jhenness@bidmc.harvard.edu

© Springer Nature Switzerland AG 2020   55
R. K. Garg et al. (eds.), *Handbook of Inpatient Endocrinology*,
https://doi.org/10.1007/978-3-030-38976-5_6

Physiologic Causes of Variations in TSH Levels in Asymptomatic Patients

Thyroid stimulating hormone (TSH) levels can vary up to 40–50% within a single day. Levels are typically lowest in the late afternoon and highest at bedtime. Normal ranges for TSH laboratory values are also determined based on where 95% of TSH values fall within a carefully screened population of healthy euthyroid volunteers. This means that 5% of people with normal thyroid function could still have TSH values that are considered abnormal. Also, these normal ranges can differ based on which reference population was studied. This chapter will give an overview of the different causes of abnormal serum TSH values not due to primary thyroid dysfunction (several of which are outlined in Fig. 6.1).

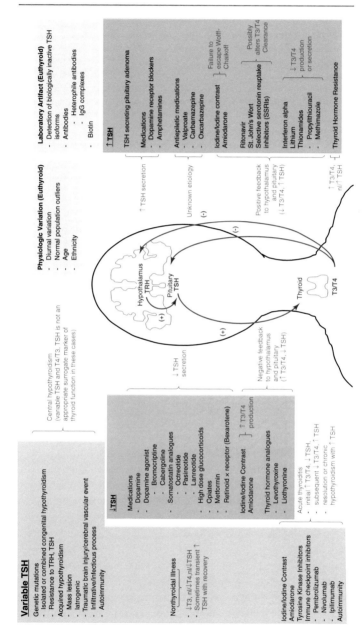

Fig. 6.1 Causes of abnormal serum TSH values not due to primary thyroid dysfunction. This figure demonstrates the normal hypothalamic-pituitary-thyroid axis. Thyrotropin-releasing hormone (TRH) is secreted by the hypothalamus that provides positive feedback to the pituitary that secretes thyroid stimulating hormone (TSH). TSH provides positive feedback to the thyroid gland causing increased production of thyroxine (T4) and triiodothyronine (T3) that both in turn provide negative feedback to the hypothalamus and pituitary. Causes of TSH abnormalities discussed in this book chapter are grouped as those that cause elevated TSH, decreased TSH, and variable TSH levels

←——————————————————————————————

Age can also affect TSH values with an estimated 0.3 mIU/L increase in value for every 10-year increase in age after 30–39 years old. TSH normal ranges can also vary based on ethnicity. In the NHANES III reference population study, African Americans aged 30–39 years old had the lowest TSH values, while Mexican Americans that were 80 years or older had the highest TSH values.

Laboratory Detection of Isoforms or Assay Interference Leading to Abnormal TSH Values in Patients Who Are Asymptomatic

Issues with laboratory detection of TSH levels can lead to abnormal values in a euthyroid patient. Several TSH isoforms can be expressed in humans that are not biologically active. Some laboratory assays may detect these isoforms leading to the reporting of abnormal TSH values that, however, do not correlate with hypothalamic-pituitary-thyroid dysfunction. Antibodies can also interfere with immunoassays used for the detection of TSH levels. Patients with high heterophile antibodies (HAb) can have falsely elevated levels. Manufactures have refined their assays to overcome this issue, but a small percentage of patients can still have high enough titers to cause interference. The most common heterophile antibodies in humans are those targeting animal antigens, specifically human anti-mouse antibodies (HAMA). Human antibodies targeting human antigens, such as rheumatoid factor, can also interfere. Suspicion should be raised in patients that have a clinical picture inconsistent with their lab values. People at high risk for development of these antibodies are those who have had recent vaccines, blood transfusions, and monoclonal antibody treatments, veterinarians, or those who have jobs that require frequent animal contact. If there is suspicion that there is a heterophile antibody, the TSH can be measured with a different manufacturer's assay.

The presence of TSH autoantibodies can cause TSH immunoglobulin G (IgG) complexes that also interfere with TSH immunoassays. This could lead to either falsely elevated or lower TSH values. These autoantibodies are immunoreactive, causing the erroneous lab values, but are not biologically active and therefore do not cause pituitary-thyroid axis dysfunction. There are assays available for removal of these IgG complexes prior to processing the serum sample.

High-dose oral biotin supplementation (>5000–10,000 μg daily) can also cause interference with the detection assays of TSH, total thyroxine (T4), and total triiodothyronine (T3). It can have a negative effect on TSH and positive effect on T3 and T4, biochemically mimicking thyrotoxicosis. Clinicians should ask about biotin supplementation so that biotin interference can be considered if the labs are inconsistent with the clinical picture. Biotin supplementation can be held prior to the blood draw to prevent interference, and the literature regarding the duration of holding biotin varies from at least 2 days to 7 days.

Medications That Can Affect TSH Levels

Medications, some of which are detailed in Table 6.1, can also affect TSH secretion and/or interrupt the hypothalamic-pituitary-thyroid axis. Often, abnormal TSH levels due to medications will normalize once the offending agent is stopped. However, some patients may require long-term antithyroidal treatment or thyroid hormone replacement therapy due to persistent thyroid dysfunction. Of note, there are several medications including iodine, iodine contrast agents, and amiodarone that can cause both hypothyroidism and thyrotoxicosis. These medications typically cause

Table 6.1 Medications that affect thyroid stimulating hormone (TSH)

Low TSH
Dopamine
Dopamine agonists
Bromocriptine
Cabergoline
Somatostatin analogues
Octreotide
Pasireotide
Lanreotide
Glucocorticoids
Opiates
Retinoid X receptor (i.e., bexarotene)
Metformin
Thyroid hormone analogues
High TSH
Dopamine receptor blockers
Amphetamines
Ritonavir
St. John's wort
Selective serotonin reuptake inhibitors (SSRIs)
Thionamides (i.e., antithyroid medications)
Propylthiouracil
Methimazole
Lithium
Antiepileptic medications
Valproate
Carbamazepine
Oxcarbazepine
Interferon alpha
High or low TSH
Immune checkpoint inhibitors
Pembrolizumab
Nivolumab
Ipilimumab

Table 6.1 (Continued)

Tyrosine kinase inhibitors
Amiodarone
Iodine/iodine contrast agents

Table derived in part from Table 10 of Garber JR, Cobin RH, Gharib H, Hennessey JV, Klein I, Mechanick JI, et al. Clinical practice guidelines for hypothyroidism in adults: cosponsored by the American Association of Clinical Endocrinologists and the American Thyroid Association. Endocr Pract Off J Am Coll Endocrinol Am Assoc Clin Endocrinol. 2012:18(6);988–1028. See Suggested Reading

thyroid dysfunction in patients who already have underlying thyroid disease or who have the propensity to develop dysfunction (i.e., antithyroid antibody positivity or nodular goiter). The development of hypo- or hyperfunction is dictated by the underlying thyroid disorder.

Medications Associated with Low TSH Levels

Dopamine infusions and agonists, high-dose glucocorticoids, somatostatin analogues including octreotide, oral bexarotene (a retinoid X receptor-selective ligand used to treat cutaneous T-cell lymphoma), metformin, and opiates have been linked to inhibition of TSH release and therefore low TSH levels. Thyroid hormone medications, including liothyronine (LT3) and levothyroxine (LT4), also lower TSH due to hypothalamic-pituitary suppression. Iodine, iodine contrast agents, and amiodarone (which is rich in iodine) can cause hyperthyroidism due to increased thyroid hormone synthesis resulting in a low TSH. The normal thyroid gland has mechanisms to prevent increased thyroid hormone production when there is excess substrate (i.e., iodine) and prevent hyperthyroidism. However, in patients who have autonomous function of the whole or part of the thyroid gland (i.e., with Graves' disease or toxic nodule), these mechanisms may be bypassed and lead to hyperthyroidism with exposure to increased iodine. Amiodarone can also cause hyperthyroidism through the mechanism outlined above due to its high iodine content. This is known as type 1 amiodarone-induced thyrotoxicosis (AIT). Type 2 AIT is a destructive thyroiditis that leads to excessive release of T3 and T4. The thyrotoxicosis can resolve or persist and eventually lead to long-term hypothyroidism.

Medications Associated with High TSH Levels

Medications including dopamine receptor blockers and amphetamines have been linked with increased TSH secretion and therefore a high TSH. Other medications such as ritonavir, St. John's wort, and selective serotonin uptake inhibitors (SSRIs) could affect the clearance of T3 and T4 leading to elevated TSH levels. Patients on long-term lithium are also at increased risk for development of hypothyroidism. This increased risk is thought to be due to decreased T4 and T3 secretion or due to a thyroiditis that may be transient. Other antiepileptic medications including valproate, carbamazepine, and oxcarbazepine have been associated with increased risk of hypothyroidism but with unclear mechanism. Interferon alpha, a treatment for hepatitis C, has been associated with hypothyroidism likely due to a destructive thyroiditis that can lead initially to transient hyperthyroidism, then to hypothyroidism, and eventually to either resolution or permanent hypothyroidism. Thionamides, used as antithyroid therapy in acute thyrotoxicosis, also causes hypothyroidism and an elevated TSH due to the blocking of thyroid hormone synthesis.

Iodine, iodine contrast agents, and amiodarone can enhance the inhibitory effect iodine has on the thyroid gland and cause hypothyroidism. As discussed above, the thyroid gland can transiently decrease thyroid hormone synthesis when there is excess iodine. This prevents the development of hyperthyroidism and is known as the Wolff-Chaikoff effect. Eventually, however, the thyroid gland will return to normal function and "escape" the Wolff-Chaikoff effect. In thyroid glands that are already damaged by preexisting autoimmune thyroiditis, the gland may not escape from the Wolff-Chaikoff effect leading to persistent hypothyroidism.

Immune Checkpoint Inhibitor Effects on TSH in Patients Treated with These Therapies

Immune checkpoint inhibitors used for cancer therapy, including anti-programed cell death protein 1 (anti PD-1) immunotherapy pembrolizumab and nivolumab and cytotoxic T-lymphocyte-associated antigen (CTLA-4) therapy with ipilimumab, have been linked with thyroid dysfunction. Clinically, patients can present with thyrotoxicosis due to thyroiditis (initially low TSH and elevated T4 that can resolve or progress to overt hypothyroidism). Patients who already have hypothyroidism can develop worsening of their hypothyroidism (elevated TSH with low T4) requiring higher doses of thyroid hormone replacement. Patients can also develop centrally mediated hypothyroidism that usually occurs with panhypophysitis. This diagnosis is made with a low free T4 levels. TSH levels can be low, inappropriately normal, or elevated. Patients with transient thyroiditis typically do not require treatment therapy. A short course of beta-blockers can be considered when there are significant clinical symptoms of thyrotoxicosis, but this is typically not required. Patients who develop overt hypothyroidism or panhypophysitis will need long-term thyroid hormone supplementation.

Tyrosine Kinase Inhibitor Effects on TSH in Patients Treated with These Therapies

Tyrosine kinase inhibitors (TKI) have been linked to hypothyroidism in euthyroid patients causing an elevated TSH. In patients who already have hypothyroidism, there can be increasing thyroid hormone replacement therapy requirements. This could be due to a transient destructive thyroiditis similar to the immune checkpoint inhibitors or possibly due to altered set points in the hypothalamic-pituitary-thyroid axis.

Nonthyroidal Illness

Serum TSH can be suppressed in patients with acute illnesses, especially those that are hospitalized and in the intensive care units. There is a distinctive pattern of serum thyroid hormone level derangements that is known as nonthyroidal illness syndrome. It is also referred to in the literature as sick euthyroid and low T3 syndrome. This entity has been described in healthy fasting patients as well as in a wide range of patients with acute and chronic illnesses including starvation, infection, trauma, surgery, sepsis, heart disease, cerebral vascular accidents, renal failure, and malignancy. It is believed that these changes help reduce energy expenditure and cellular catabolism which could have protective effects while fasting. It is unclear if these changes are an adaptive or maladaptive process in acute illness.

Thyroid Function Tests That Are Consistent with Nonthyroidal Illness

The diagnosis of nonthyroidal illness is usually obvious in acutely ill patients. Thyroid function tests show low T3 levels. T4 levels can be normal or low. TSH is typically normal but can be low. If TSH is undetectable (<0.01 mU/L), there is an increased likelihood that the patient has true hyperthyroidism. TSH levels can rise in parallel with normalization of serum T4 and T3 levels and could suggest recovery from the pituitary-thyroid axis suppression of nonthyroidal illness. If the TSH is very elevated (> 20 mU/L), there is a far higher likelihood that the patient will have persistent hypothyroidism. Serum rT3 levels can occasionally be used to help differentiate central hypothyroidism from nonthyroidal illness since it is elevated in the latter. However, its diagnostic utility is limited since it can also be slightly elevated in patients with mild hypothyroidism.

Treatment Considerations in a Patient with Nonthyroidal Illness

Several small randomized controlled trials studied treatment of nonthyroidal illness with LT3 and/or LT4 but did not show benefit in patient outcomes. Also, theoretically, if these thyroid hormone changes are adaptive, then attempts to correct the transient low T3 state could cause harm. Current recommendations are not to treat thyroid function test abnormalities likely due to nonthyroidal illness with thyroid hormone replacement unless the patient has overt clinical signs of hypothyroidism. Thyroid function tests should be checked after sufficient time has elapsed following resolution of the illness to confirm normalization of thyroid hormone levels.

Central Hypothyroidism Is Associated with Variable TSH Levels

Central hypothyroidism is characterized by an impaired TSH response. This can be caused by defects in thyrotropin-releasing hormone (TRH) – including defects in the TRH receptor – or in defects in TSH. These defects can either be due to congenital or acquired causes. Most congenital causes are due to genetic mutations and can lead to isolated central hypothyroidism or combined pituitary hormone deficiencies. With the advent of newborn screening, these are usually diagnosed during infancy. Acquired causes are typically due to processes that disrupt or destroy TRH producing cells in the hypothalamus or TRH sensing cells in the pituitary due to invasive or compressive lesions, trauma, vascular accidents, autoimmune or infectious diseases, infiltrative processes, or iatrogenic causes. Acquired causes typically lead to combined pituitary hormone deficiencies, and isolated central hypothyroidism is less common. Some of the causes of central hypothyroidism are detailed in Table 6.2. In these patients, the TSH level can either be high or low or even appear normal. However, the peripheral thyroid hormone levels (including free T4 and total T3) will be low.

Table 6.2 Causes of central hypothyroidism

Genetic causes (gene mutations)
Isolated central hypothyroidism
TSHB
TRHR
TSHR
IGSF1
TBL1X
Combined congenital hypothyroidism
LHX3, LHX4
HESX1
SOX3
OTX2
PROP1
POU1F1
LEPR
Acquired causes
Mass lesion
Pituitary adenoma (functional/nonfunctional)
Craniopharyngioma
Meningioma
Rathke's cleft cyst
Empty sella
Metastasis
Iatrogenic
Intracranial surgery
Radiation
Traumatic brain injury
Cerebral vascular events
Cerebral infarct
Intracranial hemorrhage
Sheehan's syndrome
Autoimmune disease
Lymphocytic hypophysitis
Polyglandular autoimmune disease
Infiltrative process
Sarcoidosis

Table 6.2 (Continued)

Histiocytosis X
Iron overload (hemochromatosis, blood transfusions)
Infectious diseases
Tuberculosis
Toxoplasmosis
Fungal infections

Table derived in part from Table 2 of Beck-Peccoz P, Rodari G, Giavoli C, Lania A. Central hypothyroidism - a neglected thyroid disorder. Nat Rev. Endocrinol. 2017:13;588–598. See Suggested Reading

Consider Genetic Causes of Central Hypothyroidism

The most frequent cause of inheritable *isolated* central hypothyroidism are mutations of the TSHB gene that encodes for the β-subunit of the TSH molecule. This leads to decreased levels of functional TSH and increased circulating levels of the glycoprotein hormone α-subunit (α-GSU). The α-GSU is also a subunit for follicle stimulating hormone (FSH), luteinizing hormone (LH), and human chorionic gonadotropin (hCG) and is frequently referred to as the α-subunit. A loss of function mutation in the immunoglobulin superfamily member 1 (IGSF1) gene leads to central hypothyroidism and macroorchidism. A missense mutation in the TBL1X gene is associated with central hypothyroidism and hearing loss. Mutations in pituitary transcription factors (including LHX3, LHX4, HESX1, SOX3, OTX2, PROP1, POU1F1, and LEPR genes) are the most common genetic causes of *combined* congenital hypothyroidism.

For both genetic causes of either isolated or combined congenital hypothyroidism, TSH levels can be low or normal in the setting of low free T4. These patients should be treated with levothyroxine hormone replacement. Free T4 levels should be used to monitor the adequacy of hormone replacement since TSH levels can be unreliable. Goal free T4 levels in these individuals are the same as those with central hypothyroidism, which are to be in the upper half of the normal laboratory free T4 range. It is important to remember that free T4 should be checked in the morning prior to the ingestion of a patient's levothyroxine dose because that can cause transient elevation in the free T4 level. In the case of combined congenital hypothyroidism, hormone replacement should also be initiated for any other identified pituitary hormone deficiencies.

Consider Acquired Causes of Central Hypothyroidism

Masses in the hypothalamus and/or pituitary are the most common cause of acquired central hypothyroidism. These lesions can lead to both qualitative and quantitative dysfunction of TSH. The most common masses found are nonfunctioning pituitary macroadenomas. Other lesions include craniopharyngiomas, meningiomas, Rathke's cleft cysts, metastases, as well as empty sella syndrome. Intracranial surgeries, especially for resection of a pituitary lesion, can lead to panhypopituitarism with associated central hypothyroidism. The risk of developing hypothyroidism is associated with the size and position of the tumor as well as the experience of the surgeon. Radiation therapy, especially in or around the sella, can also cause hypopituitarism with associated central hypothyroidism.

Patients with traumatic brain injury are also at risk for central hypothyroidism with an estimated disease prevalence of 15–68%. Vascular events including cerebral infarcts, subarachnoid hemorrhage, as well as Sheehan's syndrome are more rare causes of central hypothyroidism. Other less common causes of acquired central hypothyroidism include autoimmune diseases (such as lymphocytic hypophysitis which may be associated with polyglandular autoimmune disease), infiltrative processes (such as sarcoidosis, histiocytosis X, or iron overload from hemochromatosis or blood transfusions), and infectious diseases (tuberculosis, toxoplasmosis, and fungal infections).

Patients with acquired central hypothyroidism typically have low free T4. TSH can be low, inappropriately normal, or even high. High TSH levels likely reflect a qualitative defect in the circulating TSH, hence the development of hypothyroidism despite elevated TSH levels. Treatment should be with thyroid hormone replacement. Free T4 levels should be measured to monitor adequacy of hormone replacement since the TSH is unreliable. Of note, adrenal insufficiency should be ruled out in any cases where there is concern for hypopituitarism. Adrenal insufficiency should be treated prior to initiation of thyroid hormone replacement to prevent precipitation of an adrenal crisis.

Rare Causes of Abnormal TSH Levels

Resistance to TSH Causes High TSH Levels

Several point mutations in the TSH receptor gene can cause resistance to TSH. These patients typically have elevated levels of TSH with low or normal T4 and T3 concentrations. They are usually identified with newborn screens. Unlike other causes of congenital hypothyroidism, these patients do not have goiters due to the lack of TSH stimulation of the thyroid gland. Clinical symptoms and treatment are dependent on the type of mutation and percentage of functional TSH receptors present. Some patients may be euthyroid with hyperthyrotropinemia alone. Others develop severe congenital hypothyroidism requiring thyroid hormone replacement. Patients who have hyperthyrotropinemia can be differentiated from patients with autoimmune hypothyroidism because their TSH levels remain stable over time while the TSH levels change over time in autoimmune hypothyroidism. TSH levels will normalize with thyroid hormone replacement.

Resistance to TRH Is a Rare Cause of Central Hypothyroidism

A mutation in the thyrotropin-releasing hormone receptor (TRHR) has also been identified as a cause of isolated central hypothyroidism. However, this TRH resistance typically does not clinically manifest until childhood or early adulthood with delayed growth. Of note, the diagnosis of TRH resistance was made in a 33-year-old woman after her second successful pregnancy. She had normal height and IQ and had no difficulties breastfeeding, and her children had normal pre- and postnatal growth without thyroid hormone supplementation. TSH levels are typically normal, but there is a blunted TSH response to an infusion of thyrotropin-releasing hormone (TRH).

Resistance to Thyroid Hormone Is a Rare Cause of Abnormal TSH Levels

There are also mutations associated with dysfunction of thyroid hormone action. This resistance to thyroid hormone can be caused by malfunction of the thyroid hormone nuclear receptors, cell membrane transport of the hormone, or hormone metabolism. The most common mutation is associated with THRB which encodes for thyroid hormone receptor β. There is phenotypic variability even in patients with the same mutation. Typically in these syndromes, free T4 and T3 are high with normal or slightly elevated TSH. Patients can have goiters or develop attention deficit disorder and tachycardia. However, some may not have obvious symptoms of clinical thyrotoxicosis. Patients typically do not require thyroid hormone treatment because they will compensate for the insensitivity with increased T4 and T3 production. The most important thing to avoid in these patients is surgical thyroidectomy or radioactive iodine ablation of the thyroid. Mutation of the THRA gene that encodes for thyroid hormone receptor alpha is associated with low free T4, normal or slightly elevated T3, and normal TSH. The TSH is normal because the beta receptors that control TSH output remain intact. Clinically, patients exhibit signs of hypothyroidism in the peripheral tissues. These can lead to significant bony abnormalities, gastrointestinal tract dysmotility, bradycardia, and mental disabilities.

Consider TSH Secreting Tumor as a Rare Cause of High TSH and High Peripheral Thyroid Hormones

TSH secreting tumors are a very rare cause of hyperthyroidism. They represent 0.5–3% of functional pituitary adenomas, even though this could be an underestimation, and they are typically benign. Patients are usually diagnosed in their fifth to sixth decades. The majority of the lesions only secrete intact TSH, but they can also secrete growth hormone or prolactin. Sometimes there is also increased α-GSU (α-subunit). Patients develop clinical symptoms of hyperthyroidism. If it is a macroadenoma, compressive symptoms including headache and visual field defects can develop as well as adrenal and gonadal axis dysfunction. In patients who co-secrete growth hormone or prolactin, the development of acromegaly or galactorrhea may be seen.

Labs are consistent with elevated levels of T4 and T3. TSH can be inappropriately normal or mildly elevated. Patients should also be screened for hyper- and hyposecretion of other pituitary hormones, and α-GSU levels should be checked. MRI of the pituitary is recommended for imaging. Once the diagnosis of a mass is made, the patient should be evaluated by neurosurgery for resection. Interval treatment prior to surgery for hyperthyroid symptoms can include the use of beta-blockers. Somatostatin analogues or dopamine agonists can also be used for lesions that co-secrete growth hormone and prolactin.

Suggested Reading

Barroso-Sousa R, Barry WT, Garrido-Castro AC, Hodi FS, Min L, Krop IE, et al. Incidence of Endocrine Dysfunction Following the Use of Different Immune Checkpoint Inhibitor Regimens: A Systematic Review and Meta-analysis. JAMA Oncol. 2018;4(2):173–82.

Beck-Peccoz P, Rodari G, Giavoli C, Lania A. Central hypothyroidism - a neglected thyroid disorder. Nat Rev Endocrinol. 2017;13:588–98.

Bonomi M, Busnelli M, Beck-Peccoz P, Costanzo D, Antonica F, Dolci C, et al. A Family with Complete Resistance to Thyrotropin-Releasing Hormone. N Engl J Med. 2009;360(7):731–4.

Demir K, van Gucht ALM, Büyükinan M, Çatlı G, Ayhan Y, Baş VN, et al. Diverse Genotypes and Phenotypes of Three Novel Thyroid Hormone Receptor-α Mutations. J Clin Endocrinol Metab. 2016;101(8):2945–54.

Estrada JM, Soldin D, Buckey TM, Burman KD, Soldin OP. Thyrotropin isoforms: implications for thyrotropin analysis and clinical practice. Thyroid. 2014;24(3):411–23.

Fliers E, Bianco AC, Langouche L, Boelen A. Endocrine and metabolic considerations in critically ill patients 4. Lancet Diabetes Endocrinol. 2015;3(10):816–25.

Garber JR, Cobin RH, Gharib H, Hennessey JV, Klein I, Mechanick JI, et al. Clinical practice guidelines for hypothyroidism in adults: cosponsored by the American Association of Clinical Endocrinologists and the American Thyroid Association. Endocr Pract. 2012;18(6):988–1028.

Piketty M-L, Polak M, Flechtner I, Gonzales-Briceño L, Souberbielle J-C. False biochemical diagnosis of hyperthyroidism in streptavidin-biotin-based immunoassays: the problem of biotin intake and related interferences. Clin Chem Lab Med. 2017;55(6):780–8.

Refetoff S, Weiss RE, Usala SJ. The syndromes of resistance to thyroid hormone. Endocr Rev. 1993;14(3):348–99.

Tenenbaum-Rakover Y, Almashanu S, Hess O, Admoni O, Hag-Dahood Mahameed A, Schwartz N, et al. Long-term outcome of loss-of-function mutations in thyrotropin receptor gene. Thyroid. 2015;25(3):292–9.

Management of a Hospitalized Patient with Thyroid Dysfunction

7

Megan Ritter and James V. Hennessey

Contents

Abbreviations

MMI Methimazole
NPO Nil per os
PO   Per os

M. Ritter (✉)
Weill Cornell Medicine, New York Presbyterian, New York, NY, USA
e-mail: mer9114@med.cornell.edu

J. V. Hennessey
Beth Israel Deaconess Medical Center, Harvard Medical School,
Division of Endocrinology, Diabetes and Metabolism,
Boston, MA, USA
e-mail: jhenness@bidmc.harvard.edu

© Springer Nature Switzerland AG 2020   73
R. K. Garg et al. (eds.), *Handbook of Inpatient Endocrinology*,
https://doi.org/10.1007/978-3-030-38976-5_7

PTU   Propylthiouracil
T₃   Triiodothyronine
T₄   Thyroxine
TSH   Thyroid stimulating hormone

Hyperthyroidism

Antithyroid Medications

Thyroid hormone affects virtually all organ systems. Thyroxine, or T4, can be viewed as the prohormone, while triiodothyronine, or T_3, is the active form of thyroid hormone. Thyrotoxicosis can be manifested in many ways, including atrial fibrillation, weight loss, neuropsychiatric symptoms, or muscle weakness. The consequences of untreated hyperthyroidism include osteoporosis as well as frank thyroid storm which can lead to cardiovascular collapse and death. Further, untreated hyperthyroidism is associated with an increase in mortality, whereas treated hyperthyroidism negates this increase in risk. Longer duration of TSH suppression is associated with an increased hazard of mortality as well. Thus, it is prudent in both the outpatient and inpatient setting to establish the etiology of and to manage hyperthyroidism.

The 2016 American Thyroid Association guidelines recommend methimazole (MMI) as the first-line antithyroid drug except during the first trimester of a hyperthyroid woman's pregnancy when propylthiouracil (PTU) should be considered. PTU can also be used in select situations including MMI allergy or thyroid storm. Additional options for the treatment of hyperthyroidism include radioactive iodide or thyroidectomy and are tailored to patient preference in addition to concurrent medical conditions, including pregnancy or heart failure. It is reasonable to continue ambulatory doses of MMI or PTU upon hospital admission in patients who can continue to take medications orally, have no contraindications to continuing the medication, and are well-controlled outside the hospital.

Situations may arise where oral medications cannot be continued upon a patient's admission to the inpatient setting. The table reviews alternative methods physicians have used to administer antithyroid medications. Studies range from healthy volunteers without thyroid dysfunction to case reports of critically ill patients with thyroid disease (Tables 7.1 and 7.2).

These studies show that rectal administration of PTU and MMI in either enema or suppository is readily absorbed and well-tolerated for up to several days' duration. Several options exist for making a rectal application of MMI or PTU. Pharmacy availability of the different materials will determine which formulation is ultimately used to treat an individual patient. Further, although suppositories might be better tolerated based on smaller size and potentially higher degree of retention, enemas have been shown to have more rapid and robust absorption.

Intravenous (IV) medications can be advantageous when both oral and rectal administrations of medications are not possible. Given PTU's properties, methimazole has more commonly been used as an intravenous medication. Although the use of these medications IV is not widespread, the above case studies support that they can be administered IV in a safe and an effective manner.

Beta-Adrenergic-Blocking Drugs

Beta-blockers are useful in managing symptoms related to hyperthyroidism and are important initial tools in the treatment of all forms of hyperthyroidism, while diagnosis is established and control of thyroid hormone levels is being established. Atenolol, esmolol, propranolol, and metoprolol are commonly used beta-blockers but others exist. Intravenous formulations of beta-blockers are generally readily available. No studies have been found comparing efficacy of IV propranolol, IV esmolol, or IV metoprolol in hyperthyroid patients.

Pharmacokinetics of both IV esmolol and IV propranolol have been studied. IV esmolol has an elimination half-life of 2 minutes and a duration of action of 9 minutes. IV propranolol has an elimination half-life of 10 minutes and a duration of action of 2.3 hours.

Table 7.1 Alternative strategies for methimazole administration

Dose	Preparation	Patient and study characteristics	Source
(a) Intravenous administration			
10–30 mg q 6–12 hours	500 mg of MMI *USP* powder reconstituted with pH-neutral 0.9% sodium chloride to attain 10 mg MMI/mL was filtered through a 0.22 μm filter. Two mL aliquots were transferred into 10 mL sterile vials and refrigerated. MMI was pushed intravenously over 2 minutes then followed by a normal saline flush	1. A 76-year-old man with biochemical hyperthyroidism and an ileus and *Clostridium difficile* diarrhea treated with IV MMI 10 mg every 12 hours, increased to 10 mg every 8 hours. Serum FT_4 decreased from 2.9 ng/dL to 2.1 ng/dL 2. A 42-year-old male with end-stage liver disease had recurrent gastrointestinal bleeding. He was treated with IV MMI for 1 week (tapered from 30 mg IV MMI every 6 hours to 2.5 mg IV MMI every 12 hours); serum FT_4 decreased from 5.6 ng/dL to 1.6 ng/dL	Hodak SP, Huang C, Clarke D, Burman KD, Jonklaas J, Janicic-Kharic N. Intravenous methimazole in the treatment of refractory hyperthyroidism. Thyroid. 2006;16(7):691–695

10 mg, one-time dose	MMI powder was dissolved in 1 mL physiologic salt solution. Solution was enclosed in ampule and autoclaved to sterilize	Normal and hyperthyroid patients were given a one-time dose There was no difference in pharmacokinetics of MMI between normal and hyperthyroid patients	Okamura Y, Shigemasa C, Tatsuhara T. Pharmacokinetics of methimazole in normal subjects and hyperthyroid patients. Endocrinol Jpn. 1985;33(5):605–615
(b) Rectal administration			
60 mg (one-time dose)	*Suppository:* 1200 mg MMI dissolved in 12 mL of water. Two drops Span 80® added to 52 mL cocoa butter. Solution placed in 2.6 mL suppository molds	One suppository was administered to euthyroid volunteers Peak serum MMI levels were not statistically different among groups. No thyroid outcomes were measured	Nabil N, Miner DJ, Amatruda JM. Methimazole: an alternative route of administration. J Clin Endocrinol Metab. 1982;54(1):180–181

Table 7.2 Alternative strategies for PTU administration

Dose	Preparation	Patient characteristics	Source
(a) Intravenous			
50 mg	PTU tablets were dissolved in alkalinized 0.9% normal saline and then administered in 50 mg/mL doses	A 27-year-old woman, with a history of multiple small bowel resections, developed hyperthyroidism secondary to Graves' disease	Gre Gregoire, G. Presented at the 77th annual meeting of the Endocrine Society
(b) Rectal			
400 mg (one-time dose)	*Suppository*: 200 mg of PTU dissolved into an unspecified amount of polyethylene glycol base. *Enema*: eight, 50 mg tablets of ground PTU dissolved in 90 mL sterile water	Patients with biochemical hyperthyroidism were given a one-time dose of either suppository or enema before transition to PO medication. Enema group was found to have higher peak levels of PTU. Concentration rT_3 increased and serum FT_3 decreased	Jongjaroenprasert W, Akarawut W, Chantasart D, Chailurkit L, Rajatanavin R. Rectal Administration of Propylthiouracil in hyperthyroid patients: comparison of suspension Enema and suppository form. Thyroid. 2004;12(7):627–631

400 mg q 6 hours	*Suppository*: 50 mg PTU tablets solubilized in light mineral oil. This was mixed in 36 g of cocoa butter solid suppository base. One gram suppository molds were made	A 47-year-old male with thyrotoxicosis and a perforated gastric ulcer. Serum FT_4 levels decreased from 5.6 to 2.5 ng/dL during 5 days of administration	Zweig S, Schlosser JR, Thomas SA, Levy CJ, Fleckman AM. Rectal administration of propylthiouracil in suppository form in patients with thyrotoxicosis and critical illness: case report and review of literature. Endocr Pract. 2006;12(1):43–47
400 mg q 6 hours	*Suppository*: eight, 50 mg PTU tables were dissolved in 60 mL Fleets' mineral oil or 60 mL Fleet's phospho soda	A 49-year-old woman with thyroid storm and perforated viscus treated with IV methylprednisolone, IV propranolol, and rectal PTU. Serum thyroxine decreased from 26 μg/dL to 8.1 μg/dL after 3 days	Walter RM Jr., Bartle WR. Rectal administration of propylthiouracil in the treatment of graves' disease. Am J Med. 1990;88(1):69–70

PTU is largely insoluble at physiologic pH, so its use intravenously is limited but has been reported

Onset of drug action is similar. Given the rapidly changing clinical course that often accompanies thyrotoxicosis, IV esmolol may be beneficial since effects wear off rapidly; however, caution should be observed since a drop in blood pressure may occur. Propranolol does have the effect of reducing plasma T3 concentrations. However, the clinical relevance of this is uncertain as the doses of propranolol that cause reductions in T3 are larger than doses used clinically. Metoprolol can be dosed intravenously every 4–6 hours for heart rate control and is beta-1 selective, which can be beneficial in patients with heart failure. Ultimately, esmolol, propranolol, and metoprolol are all viable options in managing hyperthyroidism, and the dose will be titrated according to the patient's hemodynamics.

Glucocorticoids

Glucocorticoids decrease peripheral conversion of thyroxine (T_4) to triiodothyronine (T_3) and can be used to treat thyrotoxicosis and thyroid storm. Hydrocortisone, methylprednisolone, and dexamethasone are available in intravenous forms and a review of their characteristics is discussed below (Table 7.3).

Iodine

SSKI and Lugol's solution can be used to treat thyrotoxicosis and are indicated in the treatment of thyroid storm. Inorganic iodine reduces release of preformed T_3 and T_4. Five drops of SSKI, 0.25 mL, is equivalent to 250 mg iodine and can be dosed every 6–8 hours. Five to seven drops of Lugol's solution can be used every 6–8 hours as well. SSKI has been administered rectally after diluting with 20 to 60 mL of sterile water.

Hypothyroidism

Upon admission to an inpatient setting, levothyroxine (LT-4) therapy should be continued in order to maintain a patients' euthyroid state. It is commonly known that LT-4 absorption is impaired by

Table 7.3 Characteristics of glucocorticoids

	Equivalent dose (mg)	Anti-inflammatory activity	Mineralocorticoid activity	Duration of action (hours)
Hydrocortisone	20	1	1	8–12
Prednisone*	5	4	0.8	12–36
Prednisolone	5	4	0.8	12–36
Methylprednisolone	4	5	0.5	12–36
Dexamethasone	0.75	25	0	36–72

*Prednisone is administered orally and there is no intravenous form
Adapted From: Goodman LS, Brunton LL, Chabner B, Knollmann BC, editors. Goodman & Gilman's pharmacological basis of therapeutics. 13th ed. New York: McGraw-Hill; 2017

food and that the ideal way to ensure a stable degree of absorption from day-to-day is to take LT-4 fasting, at least 60 minutes prior to eating or 3–4 hours after eating. There are several medications known to impair levothyroxine absorption. Clinically, this can be manifested as an increase in TSH and development of a frank hypothyroid state after previously being euthyroid. Medications that can reduce PO LT-4 absorption include calcium carbonate, cholestyramine, aluminum hydroxide, sevelamer, raloxifene, and ferrous sulfate. The data regarding proton pump inhibitor (PPI) impact on PO LT-4 absorption is mixed. But, LT-4 dosing should be separated from any PPI administration since increases in TSH with initiation of PPI therapy have been reported. During a patient's hospitalization, LT-4 should not be combined with any other medications at time of administration and should be given while the patient is fasted (i.e., first thing in the morning or 3–4 hours after the last PO intake).

In contrast to treating NPO hyperthyroid patients, treating NPO hypothyroid patients is simpler. Options for treating NPO patients with hypothyroidism include intravenous LT-4 or sublingual LT-4, or subcutaneous and intramuscular LT-4 injections have been reported in the literature, but these are not approved routes for administration. Pharmacokinetic studies of intramuscular LT-4 have not been done, so it is difficult to determine if a dose change is required.

The absorption of oral LT-4 is incomplete; thus, transitioning to intravenous dosing can be challenging. Understanding oral absorption can help better tailor intravenous LT-4 dosing. Hays and Nielson (1994, see suggested readings) analyzed LT-4 absorption in patients based on age. In subjects between 21-year-olds and 69-year-olds, PO LT-4 absorption did not differ with age and was $69.3 \pm 11.9\%$. In subjects over 70 years, PO LT-4 absorption was reduced at $62.8 \pm 13.5\%$ with $p < 0.001$. When transitioning to intravenous LT-4, a dose reduction of 30% for patients less than 70 years and 40% in patients over 70 years is reasonable. The American Thyroid Association recommends a dose reduction of 25% in a patient's LT-4 dose in hospitalized patients with compromised enteral absorption. If intravenous LT-4 therapy is prolonged, reassessing thyroid function may be indicated.

Levothyroxine can be prepared in liquid and soft gel forms. The liquid form of LT-4 is LT-4 dissolved in glycerol and ethanol, while soft gel formulation LT-4 is dissolved in glycerin surrounded by a layer of gelatin. Both formulations have been used to treat hypothyroidism, particularly in patients with malabsorption.

Some patients with hypothyroidism are treated with a combination of levothyroxine and liothyronine. It is reasonable to continue an oral outpatient regimen in a euthyroid patient with an intact gastrointestinal tract and no impairments in absorption. Liothyronine is also available intravenously and can be used in the treatment of myxedema coma. There is extremely limited data on intravenous liothyronine in hospitalized patients who are NPO, so it would be reasonable to continue an outpatient regimen or transition to LT-4 monotherapy at an appropriate increased dose.

Suggested Reading

Burch HB, Cooper DS. Management of graves disease: a review. JAMA. 2015;314(23):2544.

Carroll R, Matfin G. Review: endocrine and metabolic emergencies: thyroid storm. Ther Adv Endocrinol Metab. 2010;1(3):139–45.

De Leo S, Lee SY, Braverman LE. Hyperthyroidism. Lancet. 2016;388(10047):906–18.

Goodman LS, Brunton LL, Chabner B, Knollmann BC, editors. Goodman & Gilman's pharmacological basis of therapeutics. 13th ed. New York: McGraw-Hill; 2017.

Hays MT, Nielsen KRK. Human thyroxine absorption: age effects and methodological analyses. Thyroid. 1994;4(1):55–64.

Hodak SP, Huang C, Clarke D, Burman KD, Jonklaas J, Janicic-Kharic N. Intravenous methimazole in the treatment of refractory hyperthyroidism. Thyroid. 2006;16(7):691–5.

Jongjaroenprasert W, Akarawut W, Chantasart D, Chailurkit L, Rajatanavin R. Rectal Administration of propylthiouracil in hyperthyroid patients: comparison of suspension enema and suppository form. Thyroid. 2004;12(7):627–31.

Jonklaas J, Bianco AC, Bauer AJ, Burman KD, Cappola AR, Celi FS, et al. Guidelines for the treatment of hypothyroidism: prepared by the american thyroid association task force on thyroid hormone replacement. Thyroid. 2014;24(12):1670–751.

Liwanpo L, Hershman JM. Conditions and drugs interfering with thyroxine absorption. Best Pract Res Clin Endocrinol Metab. 2009;23(6):781–92.

Nabil N, Miner DJ, Amatruda JM. Methimazole: an alternative route of administration. J Clin Endocrinol Metab. 1982;54(1):180–1.

Okamura Y, Shigemasa C, Tatsuhara T. Pharmacokinetics of methimazole in normal subjects and hyperthyroid patients. Endocrinol Jpn. 1985;33(5):605–15.

Reilly CS, Wood M, Koshakji RP, Wood AJ. Ultra-short-acting beta-blockade: a comparison with conventional beta-blockade. Clin Pharmacol Ther. 1985;38(5):579–85.

Ross DS, Burch HB, Cooper DS, Greenlee MC, Laurberg P, Maia AL, et al. American thyroid association guidelines for diagnosis and management of hyperthyroidism and other causes of thyrotoxicosis. Thyroid. 2016;26(10):1343–421.

Walter RM Jr, Bartle WR. Rectal administration of propylthiouracil in the treatment of graves' disease. Am J Med. 1990;88(1):69–70.

Wiersinga WM. Propranolol and thyroid hormone metabolism. Thyroid. 1991;1(3):273–7.

Zweig S, Schlosser JR, Thomas SA, Levy CJ, Fleckman AM. Rectal administration of propylthiouracil in suppository form in patients with thyrotoxicosis and critical illness: case report and review of literature. Endocr Pract. 2006;12(1):43–7.

Perioperative Management of Patients with Hyperthyroidism or Hypothyroidism Undergoing Nonthyroidal Surgery

8

Catherine J. Tang
and James V. Hennessey

Contents

C. J. Tang (✉) · J. V. Hennessey
Beth Israel Deaconess Medical Center, Harvard Medical School,
Division of Endocrinology, Diabetes and Metabolism,
Boston, MA, USA
e-mail: ctang@bidmc.harvard.edu; jhenness@bidmc.harvard.edu

© Springer Nature Switzerland AG 2020
R. K. Garg et al. (eds.), *Handbook of Inpatient Endocrinology*,
https://doi.org/10.1007/978-3-030-38976-5_8

Assess the Preoperative Patient

- History and physical: Focus on comorbid cardiopulmonary disease and other endocrine disorders.
- Labs: thyroid function test (TFT) including TSH and free T4 if hypothyroid or TSH, free T4, and total T3 if hyperthyroid; complete blood count (CBC) and basic metabolic panel (BMP).
- Radiology: chest X-ray to look for tracheal deviation and compression.
- Other testing: indirect laryngoscopy if thyroid gland is enlarged to look for vocal cord dysfunction (if present may indicate a difficult intubation).
- Anesthesia: airway management.

Evaluate the Type of Surgery

Once a patient is determined to have a thyroid function abnormality, the next step is to assess the urgency of the surgery. If the surgery can wait until thyroid hormone levels become normal, which may take several weeks or longer, then it is considered elective. If the surgery must be done within a few days, then it is considered urgent (see Table 8.1).

The Hypothyroid Patient Undergoing Nonthyroid Surgery

Thyroid hormone acts on nearly every tissue in the body and regulates essential metabolic pathways, including energy balance, thermogenesis, normal growth, and development [1, 2]. About 90% of free thyroid hormone circulating in the blood is in the form of thyroxine (T4), which is converted to the more potent triiodothyronine (T3) by deiodinase enzymes in the target tissues. The effect of thyroid hormone on the cardiopulmonary system is the primary concern in surgical outcomes, including decreases in

Table 8.1 Summary table

Hypothyroidism		Elective surgery	Urgent surgery	Postoperative
	Subclinical hypothyroidism	Proceed	Proceed	Reassess thyroid status as clinically indicated
	Moderate hypothyroidism	Wait until euthyroid	Age <60 years and no CVD: Start PO LT4 at 1.6 mcg/kg daily at time of diagnosis Age >60 years or CVD: Start PO LT4 at 12.5–75 mcg daily at time of diagnosis	Continue PO LT4
	Severe hypothyroidism	Wait until euthyroid	Immediately start IV LT4 200–400 mcg loading dose, followed by maintenance IV given at 75% of oral dose 1.6 mcg/kg daily. If patient not responding, optional addition of IV T3 at a loading dose of 5–20 mcg, followed by a maintenance dose of 2.5–10 mcg every 8 h) to normalize thyroid function If hemodynamically unstable or pituitary-adrenal axis is unknown, start IV hydrocortisone 50–100 mg every 6–8 h *before* the administration of thyroid hormone	Switch to PO LT4 monotherapy Taper glucocorticoid as tolerated Reassess pituitary-adrenal axis outpatient

(continued)

Table 8.1 (continued)

		Elective surgery	Urgent surgery	Postoperative
Hyperthyroidism	Subclinical hyperthyroidism	Start a BB (preferably beta-1 selective blocker such as atenolol or metoprolol succinate) and proceed	Start a BB (preferably beta-1 selective blocker such as atenolol or metoprolol succinate) and proceed	Can stop BB
	Overt hyperthyroidism	Wait until euthyroid	BB + ATD ± inorganic iodine (add at least 1 h after thionamide is given) GD and unable to tolerate ATD: BB + inorganic iodine TNG and unable to tolerate ATD: BB alone If high risk for thyroid storm regardless of underlying thyroid etiology, also add glucocorticoid ± cholestyramine	Continue BB Continue thionamide Stop inorganic iodine Taper glucocorticoid over 3 postoperative days Stop cholestyramine

Abbreviations: *CVD* cardiovascular disease, *LT4* levothyroxine, *T3* triiodothyronine or liothyronine, *BB* beta-blocker, *ATD* antithyroid drug (thionamide), *GD* Graves' disease, *TNG* toxic nodular goiter, inorganic iodine – iopanoic acid, SSKI, or Lugol's solution systemic vascular resistance, cardiac output, cardiac contractility, heart rate, blood volume, and blood pressure. Clinically, this may present as hypotension, bradycardia, hypoventilation, narrowed pulse pressure, cardiomyopathy, pericardial effusion, and tamponade. Other systems can also be adversely affected, resulting in constipation (decreased gastrointestinal motility), hyponatremia (increased antidiuretic hormone), anemia, hypoglycemia, and drug toxicity (reduced renal and hepatic clearance).

However, there are no randomized controlled studies that evaluated the surgical outcomes of hypothyroid versus euthyroid patients in nonthyroidal surgeries, though there are data from retrospective and observational studies. Clinical judgment pertaining to each individual case is thus crucial.

Elective Surgery

Subclinical Hypothyroidism

Generally, if the surgery is elective, patients should be rendered euthyroid before proceeding to surgery. The exception may be subclinical hypothyroidism, where the thyroid-stimulating hormone (TSH) is elevated above reference range but typically lower than 10 μIU/ml and a normal free thyroxine level (FT4). A South Korean observational study found that subclinical hypothyroidism was associated with an increased incidence of transient postoperative atrial fibrillation (45.5% vs. 29%) in patients who underwent coronary artery bypass grafting (CABG) [3]. However, the sample size was small (N = 36 subclinical hypothyroid patients), and the subclinical hypothyroid group had a higher rate of preoperative acute myocardial infarction (within 3 months of CABG) compared with the euthyroid group, raising the possibility of acute myocardial damage that predisposed to atrial fibrillation. The study did not find any other differences in cardiopulmonary outcomes, including other types of arrhythmias, myocardial infarction, stroke, or respiratory complications. A Boston, Massachusetts, retrospective study found that patients with subclinical hypothyroidism who underwent percutaneous transluminal angioplasty (PTCA) showed no differences in success of the procedure, hospital discharge destination, hospital costs, or in-hospital mortality [4]. Given the lack of strong evidence that subclinical hypothyroidism has a significant negative impact on surgical outcomes, the clinician must consider the patient's other comorbidities and anticipate possible minor surgical complications. Thus, the decision to proceed with an elective surgery should be individualized, but generally it is reasonable to do so.

Overt Hypothyroidism

In contrast, in patients with overt hypothyroidism, where the TSH is above and the FT4 is below the reference range, elective surgery should be deferred until euthyroidism has been achieved. A retrospective study at Massachusetts General Hospital in Boston, MA, compared surgical outcomes in 40 hypothyroid patients matched with 80 euthyroid controls [5]. The hypothyroid patients had a median TSH of 99 (reference 0.5–3.5 µIU/ml) and T4 of 2.0 (reference 4.0–12.0 µg/dl). The study found that in noncardiac surgery, hypothyroid patients were more likely to have intraoperative hypotension, though it was corrected quickly with no associated myocardial infarction or cerebrovascular accident. There was no difference in rate of intraoperative arrhythmias or the amount of blood loss. Among patients undergoing cardiac surgery, hypothyroid patients were more likely to have perioperative heart failure, but no differences in myocardial infarction or arrhythmias were observed. The authors acknowledged that there might be an inherent bias in these observations in a retrospective study. Other notable findings in the hypothyroid patients included greater prevalence of postoperative gastrointestinal (constipation, ileus) and neuropsychiatric (confusion, psychosis) occurrences in hypothyroid patients. Hypothyroid subjects were also more likely to have experienced a difficult endotracheal intubation and were less likely to manifest postoperative fever in response to infection. However, there was no difference in pulmonary complications, hyponatremia, length of hospitalization, or death rates.

Another retrospective study at the Mayo Clinic in Rochester, MN, compared surgical outcomes in 59 hypothyroid patients and 59 matched euthyroid controls [6]. The study found that hypothyroid patients had more preoperative risk factors including lower hemoglobin levels and a higher rate of hypertension, but no difference in surgical outcomes were observed, including intraoperative blood pressure, arrhythmias, fluid and electrolyte imbalances, myocardial infarction, pulmonary complications, bleeding complications, sepsis, or length of hospitalization. There was a trend toward longer time to extubation in hypothyroid patients, though it was not statistically significant. Postoperative gastrointestinal and neuropsychiatric outcomes were not assessed in this study. Admittedly, these studies are older, had small sample sizes, and may therefore not conclusive. Nonetheless, if a surgery is elective, it is prudent to render the overtly hypothyroid patient euthyroid to avoid any potential perioperative complications such as intraoperative hypotension and prolonged time to extubation.

In addition to medical management, careful attention should also be paid to airway management. Obstructive goiters may be present in either hypo- or hyperthyroidism and can cause mechanical difficulties for the anesthesiologist. Retrosternal goiters may obstruct the inferior vena cava, and vocal cord dysfunction may cause a difficult intubation. For these reasons, patients with a goiter may need additional preoperative assessment including a chest X-ray to look for tracheal compression and deviation, as well as an indirect laryngoscopy to look for vocal cord dysfunction [7].

Urgent Surgery

Subclinical Hypothyroidism
In patients with subclinical hypothyroidism, it is generally fine to proceed with an urgent surgery, for the reasons stated above in "elective surgery."

Overt Hypothyroidism
However, overtly hypothyroid patients should initiate thyroxine (T4) replacement as soon as possible as to minimize the delay in proceeding with an urgent surgery. Both the American Thyroid Association (ATA) and the American Association of Clinical Endocrinologists (AACE) recommend levothyroxine (LT4) to be the drug of choice in the treatment of hypothyroidism [8, 9],

which has largely replaced the previously favored desiccated thyroid. Due to the variable bioequivalence of several levothyroxine tablet and one gelatin formulations on the market, it is best to maintain the same preparation, whether brand or generic, in order to minimize fluctuations in thyroid hormone levels. The initial LT4 dosage depends on the severity of the hypothyroidism, etiology of the hypothyroidism, age, and comorbidities. In general, a full replacement dose of 1.6 mcg/kg of actual body weight per day can be initiated in younger patients (<60 years old) who are otherwise healthy with no cardiovascular comorbidities. On the other hand, older patients (>60 years) or those with known cardiovascular disease should start at a lower dose, from 12.5 to 75 mcg daily, erring on the lower range in patients with cardiovascular disease and higher range if TSH >12 mIU/L [8, 9]. Repeat TSH monitoring should be done every 4–6 weeks. However, given that it usually takes several weeks for the TSH to normalize, it is not always necessary to wait until euthyroidism if surgery must be done urgently. As such, the surgery and anesthesia teams should anticipate possible mild to moderate perioperative complications as detailed above under "elective surgery" and prepare accordingly.

In the case of severe hypothyroidism where the patient has or is suspected to have myxedema coma, surgery should be delayed until patient is adequately treated. However, if surgery is urgent and cannot be delayed, then intravenous (IV) replacement with LT4 should be instituted immediately, at a loading dose of 200–400 mcg, with the lower end of the range for patients who are older and have smaller body habitus and in the presence of cardiovascular comorbidities. Maintenance levothyroxine should be given intravenously at 75% (approximately the fraction of oral LT4 that is absorbed) of the oral dosing at 1.6 mcg/kg of body weight per day. The administration of intravenous liothyronine (T3) in addition to IV LT4 is optional. The rationale is that peripheral T4 to T3 conversion is decreased in acutely ill patients, and IV T3 may accelerate clinical improvement. If used, the loading dose of IV T3 is 5–20 mcg, followed by a maintenance dose of 2.5–10 mcg every 8 h. Again, one should aim for the lower end of the range for patients who are older and have smaller body habitus and in the presence of cardiovascular comorbidities [9].

Concurrent adrenal insufficiency must be considered in myxedematous patients, and if they are hemodynamically unstable or the function of their pituitary-adrenal axis is unknown, IV stress dose corticosteroids should be given *before* the administration of thyroid hormones, to avoid the precipitation of an adrenal crisis. A typical regimen is hydrocortisone 50–100 mg every 6–8 h. Once clinical improvement ensues, LT4 can be switched to an oral formulation. Generally, T3 is not continued orally and LT4 monotherapy is preferred for maintenance. Note that even with immediate treatment, patients in myxedema coma remain high surgical risk and should have close perioperative hemodynamic monitoring. Thus, a multidisciplinary approach with the surgeon, anesthesiologist, and endocrinologist is crucial in caring for these patients who must undergo urgent surgery.

The Hyperthyroid Patient Undergoing Nonthyroid Surgery

Excess thyroid hormone produces classic features of hyperthyroidism such as weight loss, tremor, heat intolerance, and hyperactivity. In the cardiovascular system, too much thyroid hormone increases cardiac contractility, heart rate, cardiac output, and systolic blood pressure, while decreases in diastolic blood pressure and systemic vascular resistance are observed. In the pulmonary system, excess thyroid hormone increases oxygen consumption, respiratory rate, and minute ventilation while decreasing vital capacity and lung compliance. Cardiovascular symptoms can include palpitations, shortness of breath, tachycardia, widened pulse pressure, cardiac murmurs, and chest pain. Of particular interest to the anesthesiologist are atrial fibrillation, ischemic heart disease, and congestive heart failure [7].

Surgery in patients with poorly controlled thyrotoxicosis has been associated with a mortality rate as high as 20% [10], primarily due to the precipitation of thyroid storm. However, the actual surgical risk is probably lower in recent decades due to better perioperative management. Again, as in hypothyroidism, there are few randomized controlled studies that have evaluated the surgi-

cal outcomes of hyperthyroid versus euthyroid patients in nonthyroidal surgeries. Clinical judgment pertaining to each individual
case is thus crucial.

Elective Surgery

Subclinical Hyperthyroidism

Patients with subclinical hyperthyroidism, where the TSH may be
slightly suppressed but the levels of T3 and T4 are normal, can
generally proceed with an elective surgery, after the initiation of a
beta-blocker if no contraindications are evident. A randomized,
prospective Swedish study compared surgical outcomes in 30
hyperthyroid patients undergoing thyroid surgery (hemithyroid-
ectomy or subtotal resection) and preoperatively managed with
either methimazole and thyroxine or metoprolol alone [11]. The
methimazole and thyroxine group was treated for 12 weeks and
was rendered clinically and biochemically euthyroid prior to thyroid surgery. The metoprolol group was treated for 5 weeks and
remained biochemically hyperthyroid but appeared clinically
euthyroid prior to thyroid surgery. The two groups did not differ
in anesthetic or cardiovascular complications, nor did anyone suffer from thyroid storm. The authors' conclusion was that metoprolol alone may be a reasonable choice for preoperative
management for hyperthyroid patients needing thyroid surgeries,
with the advantage of a shorter preoperative treatment period and
without suffering any apparent serious complications. One limita-
tion of the study was that the dose of metoprolol was 200–400 mg
per day in divided doses, which is much higher than is typically
used today. But it is worth noting that this study particularly
looked at overtly hyperthyroid patients who underwent thyroid
surgeries to treat their hyperthyroidism, so it is likely that the dose
of beta-blocker requirement is actually much lower in subclinical
hyperthyroid patients. Although some clinicians still prefer propranolol for its reduction of peripheral T4 to T3 conversion, a
beta-1 selective blocker such as atenolol or metoprolol succinate
is probably better given its longer duration of action and greater
safety in patients with obstructive pulmonary disease. A starting

dose may be atenolol or metoprolol succinate 25–50 mg daily and uptitrate as needed for a target heart rate of less than 80 bpm.

Overt Hyperthyroidism

Because of the risk of precipitating thyroid storm, elective surgeries should always be postponed in patients with overt hyperthyroidism, until the patient is rendered euthyroid [10, 12]. Moreover, atrial fibrillation occurs in 10–15% of patients with overt hyperthyroidism with the prevalence higher in older individuals [12].

Urgent Surgery

Subclinical Hyperthyroidism

Patients with subclinical hyperthyroidism may proceed with urgent surgeries after the initiation of a beta-blocker, for reasons as discussed above.

Overt Hyperthyroidism

Overtly hyperthyroid patients should wait until euthyroid before proceeding with surgery. However, if surgery cannot wait and is urgent or emergent, immediate action must be taken to stabilize thyrotoxicosis to reduce the risk of perioperative mortality. For all thyrotoxic patients regardless of etiology, beta-blockers should be initiated immediately. Calcium channel blockers such as diltiazem and verapamil can be used if beta-blockers are contraindicated. There is no general consensus on the superiority of any particular beta-blocker, though each may offer its advantages. Nonspecific beta-blocker propranolol has the additional benefit of blocking 5′-mono deiodinase activity, thus decreasing peripheral T4 to T3 conversion at higher doses, and can be started at 40–80 mg PO every 4–8 h and titrated for a target heart rate less than 80 bpm [10]. Alternatively, beta-1 selective blocker such as atenolol or metoprolol succinate may be used, at an initial dose of 25–50 mg. Though they are longer acting than propranolol and the conventional once daily dosing is more convenient, realistically they may still need to be given twice daily due to the accelerated clearance seen in hyperthyroidism [12]. IV administration may be achieved through metoprolol tartrate, propranolol, or esmolol. Esmolol has the shortest half-life of only a few minutes and thus the advantage of fast adjustment of hemodynamic parameters; an initial loading dose is 250–500 mcg/kg, followed by maintenance infusion of 50–100 mcg/kg/min [10, 13]. Beta-blockers should be continued postoperatively in nonthyroidal surgeries, possibly in lower doses, for as long as the patient remains clinically thyrotoxic or until the underlying cause of the hyperthyroidism is addressed.

If the underlying etiology of hyperthyroidism is Graves' disease or toxic nodular goiter, thionamide therapy should be instituted as soon as an urgent nonthyroid surgery is deemed necessary. Thionamide is a class of antithyroid drugs (ATD) which includes propylthiouracil (PTU), methimazole (MMI), and carbimazole. Only PTU and MMI are available in the United States, whereas carbimazole is available in Europe and elsewhere. PTU and MMI can be given either orally or rectally. They block new thyroid hormone synthesis by inhibiting the enzyme thyroid peroxidase, which is responsible for the organification of iodine and the coupling of mono- and diiodotyrosines to make T3 and T4. Since thionamides largely affect new thyroid hormone synthesis but not secretion of preformed thyroid hormones, they usually take 3–8 weeks to achieve euthyroidism [12]. In the case of an urgent surgery that may take place within a matter of days or hours, thionamide therapy alone is not adequate, and additional treatment should be instituted to stabilize the thyrotoxicosis, which are discussed below. PTU is shorter acting and has the additional benefit of decreased T4 to T3 conversion. A typical starting dose of PTU is 100–150 mg every 6–8 h [12]. However, if the patient is severely hyperthyroid or if thyroid storm is suspected, the 2016 ATA guidelines recommend a PTU loading dose of 500–1000 mg, followed by 250 mg every 4 h [14]. MMI is longer acting and is generally preferred over PTU for its lesser degree of toxicities, except during the first trimester of pregnancy, when PTU is less teratogenic. A typical starting dose of MMI is 20–40 mg daily, though in a severely hyperthyroid patient, the dose is increased to 60–80 mg per day [14], which may be divided into two to three doses daily due to the increased clearance seen in hyperthyroidism. Both PTU and MMI have similar side effect profiles and have 50% cross-reactivity. Minor toxicities include rash, urticaria, and arthralgia, which occur in 1–5% of patients [10, 12]. A more serious complication is hepatotoxicity, which is more common in PTU (2.7%) than in MMI (0.4%), though liver failure remains rare in either (0.03–0.05%) [14]. Perhaps the most dreaded toxicity is agranulocytosis, which occurs in 0.1–0.5% of patients [10, 14], with the vast majority of cases occurring within 60–90 days of starting therapy. Although the effect is conventionally thought to be dose-related in MMI (rare at doses below 40 mg daily) but not in PTU, a more recent Danish study demonstrated that the average dose of MMI at the onset of agranulocytosis was 25 mg daily in patients with Graves' disease [15]. Postoperatively, ATD should be continued at the same dose until thyroid hormone levels are no longer elevated.

As mentioned earlier, since ATD takes 3–8 weeks to achieve euthyroidism, it alone is not sufficient in preparing a patient for urgent surgery. In such cases, inorganic iodine should be added to ATD to decrease the production of new thyroid hormone, which is also known as the Wolff-Chaikoff effect and can be seen within 24 h of administration. In addition, inorganic iodine also decreases the release of preformed thyroid hormone. A normal thyroid gland will eventually escape the Wolff-Chaikoff effect and resume thyroid hormone production, but the effect may persist in those with autoimmune thyroid disease. In contrast, a toxic nodular goiter (TNG) may use the excess iodine as substrate to make more thyroid hormone (known as the Jod-Basedow effect), further exacerbating the thyrotoxicosis [10, 12]. For this reason, while iodine can be used as monotherapy in Graves' disease, it should never be used as monotherapy in TNG. In fact, it is crucial that iodine should be given at least an hour *after* the administration of a thionamide. In this setting where thyrotoxicosis must be urgently stabilized, iodine can be administered as saturated solution of potassium iodide (SSKI) five drops (50 mg of iodide per drop) every 6 h [12, 14]. Inorganic iodine should be stopped after surgery.

Other agents that may be used in the acutely thyrotoxic patient regardless of the underlying cause in preparation of urgent surgery include glucocorticoids and cholestyramine. Glucocorticoids reduce peripheral T4 to T3 conversion within hours and can be tapered over 72 h postoperatively [10, 12]. Choice of glucocorticoids includes hydrocortisone 100 mg every 8 h, dexamethasone 2 mg every 6 h, or betamethasone 0.5 mg every 6 h, which all can be given either IV or PO (betamethasone can also be given as IM) [10, 12]. Postoperatively, glucocorticoids should be tapered over the course of 72 h [10, 12]. Cholestyramine, a bile acid sequestrant, binds to thyroid hormone in the intestine and reduces its reabsorption, thus decreasing its enterohepatic circulation. It is not a first- or second-line agent but is potentially useful in situations where it is not possible to render the patient completely euthyroid prior to surgery or if the patient is intolerant of ATD [14]. A typical dose of cholestyramine used in this setting is 4 g four times daily [12]. Cholestyramine is generally stopped postoperatively.

Patients who are intolerant of ATD and those who have Graves' disease as the underlying etiology may be treated with beta-blockers and iodine, with the addition of glucocorticoid and possibly cholestyramine if hyperthyroidism is severe. In ATD-intolerant patients whose underlying etiology is TNG, preoperative management may consist of beta-blockers alone, with the addition of glucocorticoid and possibly cholestyramine if hyperthyroidism is severe. Iodine is not used in this scenario due to concern of exacerbating thyrotoxicosis, for the reasons stated previously.

As in the case of severe hypothyroidism, patients with severe hyperthyroidism remain high surgical risk despite optimal perioperative management. A multidisciplinary approach with the surgeon, anesthesiologist, and endocrinologist is vital in the caring of these patients who require urgent surgeries, and careful attention must be paid to airway management (due to goiters, as discussed in the previous section) and hemodynamic monitoring.

References

1. Lin JZ, Martagón AJ, Cimini SL, Gonzalez DD, Tinkey DW, Biter A, et al. Pharmacological activation of thyroid hormone receptors elicits a functional conversion of white to brown fat. Cell Rep. 2015;13(8):1528–37.

2. Mullur R, Liu YY, Brent GA. Thyroid hormone regulation of metabolism. Physiol Rev. 2014;94(2):355–82.
3. Park YJ, Yoon JW, Kim KI, Lee YJ, Kim KW, Choi SH, et al. Subclinical hypothyroidism might increase the risk of transient atrial fibrillation after coronary artery bypass grafting. Ann Thorac Surg. 2009;87(6):1846–52.
4. Mantzoros CS, Evagelopoulou K, Moses AC. Outcome of percutaneous transluminal coronary angioplasty in patients with subclinical hypothyroidism. Thyroid. 1995;5(5):383–7.
5. Ladenson PW, Levin AA, Ridgway EC, Daniels GH. Complications of surgery in hypothyroid patients. Am J Med. 1984;77(2):261–6.
6. Weinberg AD, Brennan MD, Gorman CA, Marsh HM, O'Fallon WM. Outcome of anesthesia and surgery in hypothyroid patients. Arch Intern Med. 1983;143(5):893–7.
7. Farling PA. Thyroid disease. Br J Anaesth. 2000;85(1):15–28.
8. Garber JR, Cobin RH, Gharib H, Hennessey JV, Klein I, Mechanick JI, Pessah-Pollack R, Singer PA, Woeber KA, American Association of Clinical Endocrinologists and American Thyroid Association Taskforce on Hypothyroidism in Adults. Clinical practice guidelines for hypothyroidism in adults: cosponsored by the American Association of Clinical Endocrinologists and the American Thyroid Association. Endocr Pract. 2012;18(6):988–1028.
9. Jonklaas J, Bianco AC, Bauer AJ, Burman KD, Cappola AR, Celi FS, et al. Guidelines for the treatment of hypothyroidism: prepared by the American Thyroid Association task force on thyroid hormone replacement. Thyroid. 2014;24(12):1670–751.
10. Langley RW, Burch HB. Perioperative management of the thyrotoxic patient. Endocrinol Metab Clin North Am. 2003;32(2):519–34.
11. Adlerberth A, Stenstrom G, Hasselgren PO. The selective beta 1-blocking agent metoprolol compared with antithyroid drug and thyroxine as preoperative treatment of patients with hyperthyroidism. Results from a prospective, randomized study. Ann Surg. 1987;205(2):182–8.
12. Palace MR. Perioperative management of thyroid dysfunction. Health Serv Insights. 2017;10:1178632916689677.
13. Buget MI, Sencan B, Varansu G, Kucukay S. Anaesthetic management of a patient with thyrotoxicosis for nonthyroid surgery with peripheral nerve blockade. Case Rep Anesthesiol. 2016;2016:9824762.
14. Ross DS, Burch HB, Cooper DS, Greenlee MC, Laurberg P, Maia AL, et al. 2016 American Thyroid Association guidelines for diagnosis and management of hyperthyroidism and other causes of thyrotoxicosis. Thyroid. 2016;26(10):1343–421.
15. Andersen SL, Olsen J, Laurberg P. Antithyroid drug side effects in the population and in pregnancy. J Clin Endocrinol Metab. 2016;101(4): 1606–14.

Thyroid Problems Encountered Specifically in Inpatients with Cardiac Disease

9

Jeena Sandeep and James V. Hennessey

Contents

J. Sandeep (✉)
St. Elizabeth Medical Center, Department of Medicine,
Division of Endocrinology, Brighton, MA, USA
e-mail: jeena.sandeep@steward.org

J. V. Hennessey
Beth Israel Deaconess Medical Center, Harvard Medical School,
Division of Endocrinology, Diabetes and Metabolism,
Boston, MA, USA
e-mail: jhenness@bidmc.harvard.edu

© Springer Nature Switzerland AG 2020
R. K. Garg et al. (eds.), *Handbook of Inpatient Endocrinology*,
https://doi.org/10.1007/978-3-030-38976-5_9

Hyperthyroidism/Thyrotoxicosis

- Thyrotoxicosis – excessive thyroid hormone regardless of etiology – affects the cardiovascular system resulting in cardiac arrhythmias, EKG changes, congestive heart failure (CHF) and angina, and/or myocardial infarction.
- Patients with subclinical thyrotoxicosis may be asymptomatic, manifest resting tachycardia, or may develop atrial fibrillation and be at risk for embolic stroke.
- Establishing the etiology of thyrotoxicosis is critical in determining appropriate therapeutic interventions. The most common conditions are Graves' disease, toxic multinodular goiter (toxic MNG) or toxic adenoma (TA), iatrogenic thyrotoxicosis, and subacute thyroiditis (SAT).
- Amiodarone can cause either hypothyroidism or thyrotoxicosis. There are two types of amiodarone-induced thyrotoxicosis (AIT) which may be difficult to differentiate from one another.
- Diagnostic evaluation includes the history, medication (iatrogenic) and supplement ingestion (factitia), viral infection, neck pain [suggestive of subacute thyroiditis]), presence of eye and pretibial symptoms (Graves' disease), and presence of thyroid nodules (toxic nodular goiter or adenoma). Lab testing includes TSH, assessment of free thyroxine, T3 testing, thyrotropin receptor antibodies (TRab), and 123-I uptake and/or scanning.

- Treatments include beta-blockers, antithyroid drugs (methimazole generally preferred), 131-I ablation, and/or surgery. Treatment for type 1 AIT includes antithyroid drugs, potassium perchlorate (not available in the United States), or surgery, and type 2 AIT may either be observed, or if mild, may be treated with glucocorticoids, and if inadequately controlled, may require surgery.

Hypothyroidism

- Hypothyroidism may affect cholesterol metabolism and other CV risk factors such as C-reactive protein and homocysteine that may promote CAD and can also predispose patients to atrial fibrillation (Afib).
- Hypothyroidism increases systemic vascular resistance (SVR) and diminishes cardiac output, stroke volume, and heart rate resulting in lower cardiac output.
- Diminished erythropoietin production results in blood volume decrease. Capillary permeability allows pericardial and pleural effusions further compromising cardiac (tamponade) and pulmonary function.
- Prolongation of the QT interval predisposes to ventricular arrhythmia and AV nodal dysfunction.
- Diagnosis requires measurement of TSH and free T4 (FT4) levels. Overt hypothyroidism is recognized when TSH is clearly elevated (over 10 mIu/L) and FT4 is low, while subclinical hypothyroidism is characterized by a sustained TSH level between the upper reference range and 10 mIu/L and a normal FT4.
- Treatment with levothyroxine (LT4) in overt hypothyroidism improves LDL cholesterol metabolism, diastolic hypertension, and cardiac dysfunction while accelerating heart rate and delaying progression of atherosclerosis. Due to potential underlying CAD, caution in reestablishing euthyroidism may be warranted. Gradual increasing doses at intervals of 6–8 week allow equilibration of thyroid hormone levels before retesting.

- Coronary bypass surgery is generally considered safe in patients with hypothyroidism. Concerns regarding perioperative care and the risk of postoperative atrial fibrillation in hypothyroid patients undergoing cardiac surgery have been raised.

Hyperthyroidism/Thyrotoxicosis

Effects on the Cardiovascular System

Increased levels of circulating thyroid hormones alter the function of the cardiovascular system and produce significant clinical effects. Increased systolic blood pressure due to increased contractile ventricular force and decreased diastolic pressure due to lower peripheral vascular resistance result in wide pulse pressure and enhanced cardiac output. Tachycardia reflects a positive chronotropic action of thyroid hormone on the heart. Increased stroke volume and volume expansion result in increased circulating blood volume. The drop in DBP leads to activation of renin angiotensin aldosterone system increasing sodium reabsorption and consequent volume expansion. Thyroid hormone directly increases erythropoietin synthesis increasing the red cell mass increasing the preload. Resting tachycardia results from thyroid hormone acting on the sinus node to increase heart rate. The net result of decreased afterload, increased left ventricular contractility, increased preload, wide pulse pressure, and increased heart rate is an overall increase in cardiac output.

Cardiac Arrhythmias and EKG Changes

Arrhythmias include resting tachycardia and atrial fibrillation which may convert to sinus rhythm within 8–12 weeks after effective antithyroid treatment in the absence of valvular heart disease and of recent onset. EKG changes include the supraventricular arrhythmias and nonspecific ST segment and T-wave changes as well as a short PR interval due to an increased rate of conduction through the AV node.

Congestive Heart Failure (CHF) and Angina

Hyperthyroidism may cause or worsen preexisting cardiac disease by increasing myocardial oxygen demand, contractility, and heart rate. These changes may lead to silent ischemia, angina, or compensated heart failure and even endothelial dysfunction. Heart failure in the thyrotoxic patient occurs in the setting of underlying coronary heart disease and/or atrial fibrillation. Cardiac failure can occur even in young patients without known underlying heart disease suggesting a cardiomyopathy associated with thyrotoxicosis which may well be reversible. Recent reports suggest an increased prevalence of pulmonary hypertension in the setting of thyrotoxicosis suggesting that thyroid hormones increase pulmonary vascular resistance in contrast to its effects on systemic vascular resistance.

Management of Thyrotoxicosis in the Hospitalized Patient

Establishing the Etiology of Thyrotoxicosis

Symptomatic patients with thyrotoxicosis, especially patients with heart rates above 90 beats per minute, elderly patients, and patients with underlying cardiovascular disease should be treated with beta-blockers while determining the etiology of thyrotoxicosis. The most frequent endogenous diagnoses of thyrotoxicosis include Graves' disease, toxic multinodular goiter (toxic MNG) or toxic adenoma (TA), and subacute thyroiditis (SAT). Graves' disease patients may be recognized by the presence of pretibial myxedema and eye involvement. Those with toxic MNG and toxic adenoma may have a prior history of thyroid nodules. The history may point to thyroiditis as the etiology. Some may report recent viral infection followed by pain and tenderness over the thyroid or have recently given birth prior to developing thyrotoxicosis. A radioactive iodine uptake is useful to distinguish exogenous sources of thyrotoxicosis and thyroiditis from Graves' disease and toxic nodular disorders.

Iodine uptake may be near zero in exogenous thyrotoxicosis, painless, postpartum or painful subacute (deQuervains) thyroiditis. In addition, low or near zero uptake can also be seen in cases of ectopic thyroid disorders such as Struma Ovarii and after iodine contamination such as post CT with iodine contrast or while on treatment with medications such as amiodarone. Radioactive iodine uptake is typically elevated and diffuse in Graves' disease while focal nodular patterns are seen in patients with toxic nodular goiters.

Treatment Recommendations Based on Etiology

Thyrotoxicosis due to exogenous thyroid hormone application is best treated with beta-blocker and discontinuation of the thyroid hormone source. Severely toxic individuals may respond quickly to plasmapheresis. Patients with subacute thyroiditis are treated with beta-blockers, nonsteroidal anti-inflammatory drugs for pain, and if needed corticosteroids. Once Graves' disease is confirmed, treatment may include antithyroid drugs (ATDs), radioactive iodine, or surgery. Patient preference is an important factor in deciding on a treatment modality. However, patients with acute cardiopulmonary disease who are clinically unstable are usually treated with ATDs followed by radioactive iodine treatment, particularly if they are still at high surgical risk. Patients who are pregnant, lactating mothers, those with coexisting thyroid cancer, and those unable to comply with radiation safety guidelines or planning a pregnancy within 4–6 months should not receive radioactive iodine. On the other hand, definite contraindications to antithyroid medication usage and switching include major adverse reactions such as agranulocytosis and hepatotoxicity.

Methimazole is the preferred ATD with the potential exception of thyroid storm, the first trimester of pregnancy, and minor reactions to methimazole when propylthiouracil (PTU) is preferred. Starting dose of methimazole is usually 10–20 mg once daily and is titrated based on the clinical and biochemical response. PTU is shorter acting and is administered multiple times a day with starting dose from 50 to 150 mg three times daily. Patients are monitored for side effects including rash, agranulocytosis (fever, sore throat), and cholestasis (pale stools, jaundice, abdominal pain, nausea, vomiting).

Thyrotoxicosis due to toxic multinodular goiter (TMNG) or toxic adenoma (TA) should be treated with radioactive iodine or surgery. Chronic low-dose methimazole can be considered for those with contraindications to definitive treatment. In patients with cardiovascular disease or elderly patients or in situations where there is high risk of worsening of hyperthyroidism post-radioactive iodine treatment, beta-blockers should be initiated prior to administering radioactive iodine treatment.

Patients undergoing surgery for Graves' disease should be treated with beta-blockers and rendered clinically and biochemically euthyroid preoperatively with ATDs. Potassium iodide may be administered in the immediate preoperative period. If the patient needs urgent surgery, beta-blocker, ATDs, and potassium iodide should be used as long as possible to achieve or approach a euthyroid state prior to surgery.

Subclinical Hyperthyroidism

Patients with subclinical thyrotoxicosis may be asymptomatic or present with resting tachycardia or atrial fibrillation. The 10-year risk of developing atrial fibrillation in elderly patients with a TSH less than 0.1 mIU/L is three times higher compared to euthyroid patients. Elderly patients with subclinical thyrotoxicosis have an increased risk of all-cause and cardiovascular mortality, while young and middle-aged people manifest cardiac changes including increased ventricular mass and contractility and reduced diastolic function. The decision to treat subclinical hyperthyroidism is based on risk. If TSH is persistently less than 0.1 mIU/L, patients older than 65 years, patients with cardiac risk factors or disease, and those with osteoporosis should be treated. In addition, patients with clinical symptoms of hyperthyroidism and postmenopausal women who are not treated with estrogens or bisphosphonates are treated if TSH is persistently lower than

0.1 mIU/L. When TSH is less than normal but above 0.1 mIU/L, treatment would be considered for patients over 65 years of age, patients who are symptomatic, and those with cardiac disease.

Treatment with Amiodarone in Patients with Cardiac Arrhythmias

Amiodarone is iodine rich (37% by weight) and concentrates in several tissues resulting in an effective half-life of more than 50 days. Amiodarone can cause both hypothyroidism and thyrotoxicosis. There are two types of amiodarone-induced thyrotoxicosis (AIT). Type 1 AIT is a form of endogenous hyperthyroidism where there is overproduction of thyroid hormone and occurs in patients with underlying thyroid disease including Graves' or multinodular goiter. Type 1 AIT occurs more frequently in areas of iodine deficiency. Type 2 AIT is a form of thyroiditis where preformed thyroid hormone is released from the thyroid in an unregulated manner. Treatment for type 1 AIT includes antithyroidal drugs, potassium perchlorate (to block thyroidal iodine uptake), or surgery. Type 2 may be observed, and if mild, may be treated with glucocorticoids or if severe may be treated with surgery if not responsive to medical therapy. It may be difficult to differentiate type 1 from type 2 AIT, and a combination of antithyroidal drugs (MMI) and glucocorticoids is frequently used as the initial treatment. There is debate if amiodarone needs to be stopped when thyrotoxicosis occurs. As amiodarone is lipophilic and may not be cleared for 6 months or more after stopping the drug, discontinuation is not of short-term use. If treatment with amiodarone is critical to controlling the arrhythmias, amiodarone should be continued.

Hypothyroidism and Cardiac Disease

Impact of Hypothyroidism on Cardiovascular Risk Factors

Both overt and subclinical hypothyroidism (SCHypo) are associated with changes in lipid parameters and are considered risk factors for cardiovascular disease. Total LDL cholesterol and apolipoprotein B levels are adversely affected by insufficient circulating thyroid hormone as decreased expression of the hepatic LDL receptor and reduced activity of cholesterol α-monooxygenase activity diminish cholesterol clearance. Other CV risk factors such as C-reactive protein and homocysteine are also elevated in the hypothyroid state. This risk profile may lead to the progression of undiagnosed coronary artery and vascular disease in patients with hypothyroidism. Additionally, the effectiveness and safety of treatment of dyslipidemia with statin medications, specifically myopathy, may be impacted by the presence of hypothyroidism.

Cardiovascular Hemodynamics in Hypothyroidism

Systemic vascular resistance (SVR) is increased and cardiac output declines. Thyroid hormone has a direct vasodilator effect on vascular smooth muscle and indirect effect by inducing endothelium-derived nitric oxide release. Both of these actions are impaired in mild and overt hypothyroidism which results in further increase in the systemic vascular resistance. Cardiac contractility is negatively affected leading to a reduction in stroke volume and decrease in heart rate which together lead to a reduction in cardiac output. Additional changes include diminished stimulation of erythropoietin production decreasing plasma and circulating blood volume. Capillary permeability increases resulting in gravity-dependent edema and pericardial and pleural effusions which may further compromise both cardiac (tamponade physiology) and pulmonary function.

Heart Failure and Arrhythmias in Hypothyroidism

The impact of hypothyroidism on cardiac contractility may result in clinical cardiac failure, often characterized as diastolic dysfunction that results in abnormal cardiac muscle relaxation. However, heart failure caused by hypothyroidism differs physiologically from heart failure caused by non-thyroidal causes. Despite reduc-

tion in cardiac output, hypothyroid patients have normal arteriove-
nous (AV) oxygen extraction as against patients with organic heart
disease and heart failure who have increased AV oxygen extraction. Patients with hypothyroidism are able to mount cardiac
response to the exercise in terms of increasing the cardiac output
and reduction in SVR as against patients with classic CHF. In addition, signs of right heart failure are rare in hypothyroid patients,
and they are able to excrete sodium load when compared with
patients with CHF from organic heart disease. Exercise intolerance
seen in hypothyroid patients is due to weakness of skeletal muscle
and due to respiratory etiology rather than cardiac failure.

As noted above, the presence of CAD risk factors potentially
predispose these patients to atrial fibrillation (Afib) which further
compromises optimal cardiac function. Recent data indicated that
hypothyroidism may predict persistently symptomatic atrial fibrillation impacting cardiovascular outcomes. A prolonged QT interval is commonly noted in hypothyroid subjects likely indicating a
ventricular vulnerability to arrhythmia, while conduction defects
across the AV node and through the ventricles are also reported.

Amiodarone-Induced Hypothyroidism

As a result of the substantial (37% by weight) iodine content of
amiodarone, those with previously damaged thyroid glands due to
autoimmune thyroid disease or 131-I ablation for Graves' are
especially susceptible to the Wolff-Chaikoff effect, thereby
decreasing thyroid hormone production and lapse into hypothyroidism after long-term treatment. Due to its prolonged half-life
and the danger posed by the underlying arrhythmias that
amiodarone so successfully treats, discontinuation of amiodarone
is not usually undertaken as it is neither an effective solution to the
hypothyroidism nor a prudent decision from a cardiac perspective.

Diagnosis of Hypothyroidism

Diagnosis requires measurement of TSH and free T4 (FT4)
levels. There is no utility in measuring T3 or reverse T3 (rT3)
if hypothyroidism is suspected. Caution should be exercised

in interpreting TSH levels (dopamine and glucocorticoids suppress TSH) and FT4 levels (change due to non-thyroidal illness [NTI]) in acutely ill patients. Overt primary hypothyroidism is characterized as a clearly elevated TSH (greater than 10 uLU/L) and low FT4. Overt central hypothyroidism is recognized when TSH is suppressed or inappropriately normal and FT4 is below the expected range. Subclinical hypothyroidism is defined as elevation of TSH with a normal FT4. TSH elevation should be reproducible to rule out the effect of non-thyroidal illness and greater than age-adjusted expected ranges. SCHypo is seldom definitively diagnosed in hospitalized patients due to the impact of NTI on TSH levels. Antithyroid antibodies to thyroid peroxidase (TPO) or thyroglobulin (Tg-ab) are useful to document the presence of autoimmune thyroid disease, and TPO may predict an increased risk of progression to overt hypothyroidism in those with SCHypo.

Treatment of Overt Hypothyroidism

Treatment with levothyroxine (LT4) improves LDL cholesterol metabolism, diastolic hypertension, and cardiac dysfunction, accelerates heart rate, and delays the progression of atherosclerosis. Additionally, prospective data clearly demonstrate that LT4 therapy will reverse the cardiac muscle lipid accumulation and reduction in cardiac output associated with short-term overt hypothyroidism. Due to the potential presence of underlying CAD in some subjects with prolonged duration of hypothyroidism, some caution in reestablishing the euthyroid state may be warranted.

The full replacement dose of levothyroxine is generally 1.6–1.7 microgram/kg daily in patients with overt hypothyroidism. However, this recommendation varies in those with SCHypo where residual endogenous thyroxine production is present. The cardiovascular system in patients with SCHypo clearly responds positively to LT4 when TSH is greater 10 mIU/L especially in those under 65 years of age. Out of an abundance of caution, lower initial replacement doses than those employed in young adults are advisable in the elderly and those with known CVD and titrated up slowly (start low and go slow). The recommended starting dose of levothyroxine in patients above 50–60 years of age is 50 microgram daily in the absence of known CAD and in those with known cardiac issues where initial doses of 12.5–25 microgram daily are recommended. LT4 should be ingested fasting with water only 60 min before breakfast or other medications for optimal absorption. Following the institution of LT4 therapy, adequate time (4–8 weeks) should pass before reevaluation of thyroid function is carried out.

Thyroid Hormone Treatment in Cardiac Failure and Patients Undergoing Cardiac Surgery

It has long been felt that emergency coronary bypass surgery is considered safe in patients with hypothyroidism. Other reports raise concern about prolonged postoperative recovery from anesthetics, ileus, and infections going undetected due to a lack of fever as well as atrial fibrillation of hypothyroid patients undergoing cardiac surgery. Preoperatively, all patients should be treated with adequate doses of thyroid hormone. Unless there are contraindications such as bradycardia and advanced COPD, beta-blockers should also be given to reduce the risk of frequently encountered post-cardiac surgery atrial fibrillation.

In patients with heart failure and normal TSH and T4, those with a low T3 concentration had more severe heart failure as assessed by New York Heart Association criteria. Short-term treatment with T3 in patients with cardiac failure has resulted in a predictable decrease in systemic vascular resistance and subsequent improvement in cardiac output without adverse effects but is not generally suggested due to limited confirmatory data. There are no guidelines which recommend treatment with IV T3 in patients with cardiac disease undergoing bypass surgery with low T3 syndrome. Presently, we do not recommend treating patients with cardiac disease with IV T3.

Suggested Reading

Alexander EK, Pearce EN, Brent GA, Brown RS, Chen H, Dosiou C, et al. 2017 Guidelines of the American Thyroid Association for the diagnosis and management of thyroid disease during pregnancy and the postpartum. Thyroid. 2017;27(3):315–89.

Bogazzi F, Tomisti L, Bartalena L, Aghini-Lombardi F, Martino E. Amiodarone and the thyroid: a 2012 update. J Endocrinol Invest. 2012;11(5):340–8.

Burch HB, Cooper DS. Management of Graves' disease: a review. JAMA. 2015;314(23):2544–54.

De Leo S, Lee SY, Braverman LE. Hyperthyroidism. Lancet. 2016;388(10047):906–18.

Garber JR, Cobin RH, Gharib H, Hennessey JV, Klein I, Mechanick JI, American Thyroid Association Taskforce on Hypothyroidism in Adults, et al. Clinical practice guidelines for hypothyroidism in adults: cosponsored by the American Association of Clinical Endocrinologists and the American Thyroid Association. Thyroid. 2012;22(12):1200–35.

Martin SS, Daya N, Lutsey PL, Matsushita K, Fretz A, McEvoy JW, et al. Thyroid function, cardiovascular risk factors, and incident atherosclerotic cardiovascular disease: the atherosclerosis risk in communities (ARIC) study. J Clin Endocrinol Metab. 2017;102(9):3306–15.

Ross DS, Burch HB, Cooper DS, Greenlee MC, Laurberg P, Maia AL, et al. ATA hyperthyroidism management guidelines. Thyroid. 2016;26(10):1343–421.

Sun J, Yao L, Fang Y, Yang R, Chen Y, Yang K. Relationship between subclinical thyroid dysfunction and the risk of cardiovascular outcomes: a systematic review and meta-analysis of prospective cohort studies. Int J Endocrinol. 2017;2017:8130796.

Teasdale SL, Inder WJ, Stowasser M, Stanton T. Hyperdynamic right heart function in Graves' hyperthyroidism measured by echocardiography normalises on restoration of euthyroidism. Heart Lung Circ. 2017;26(6):580–5.

Udovcic M, Pena RH, Patham B, Tabatabai L, Kansara A. Hypothyroidism and the heart. Methodist Debakey Cardiovasc J. 2017;13(2):55–9. houstonmethodist.org/debakey-journal.

Severe Hypercalcemia

10

Antonia E. Stephen and Johanna A. Pallotta

Contents

A. E. Stephen
Harvard Medical School, Massachusetts General Hospital,
Department of Surgery, Boston, MA, USA
e-mail: astephen@partners.org

J. A. Pallotta (✉)
Harvard Medical School, Beth Israel Deaconess Medical Center,
Department of Medicine, Endocrinology and Metabolism,
Boston, MA, USA
e-mail: jpallott@bidmc.harvard.edu

© Springer Nature Switzerland AG 2020
R. K. Garg et al. (eds.), *Handbook of Inpatient Endocrinology*,
https://doi.org/10.1007/978-3-030-38976-5_10

Introduction

Hypercalcemia is a common clinical problem. The majority of patients with hypercalcemia are asymptomatic and are often diagnosed on routine laboratory studies. They do not typically require immediate treatment. In distinction to patients with mild hypercalcemia, patients with severe hypercalcemia are often symptomatic and usually require urgent admission and treatment. In addition to treating the acute hypercalcemia, the underlying cause must be investigated and treated when possible, to avoid ongoing or repeated episodes of severe calcium elevation. In over 90% of patients, the cause of hypercalcemia is either primary hyperparathyroidism or malignancy; other causes are far less common. The focus of this chapter is on the etiology of hypercalcemia and the presentation and treatment of severe hypercalcemia.

Etiology

The etiologies of hypercalcemia are primarily distinguished between those that are parathyroid (PTH)-dependent and those arising from non-PTH-dependent mechanisms (Table 10.1). Among all causes of hypercalcemia, hyperparathyroidism (excess PTH production) remains the most common. Included in this category are primary (adenoma, hyperplasia, or rarely carcinoma of the parathyroid glands) and tertiary hyperparathyroidism (physiologic hypertrophy of the parathyroid glands). Among non-PTH-dependent etiologies, the most common cause is hypercalcemia of malignancy. This can occur as a result of the excess production of PTH-related peptides (PTHrP), from osteolytic bone metastases, or from excess vitamin D production. Less common causes of hypercalcemia include hypervitaminosis D, also known as vitamin D intoxication, where excessive vitamin D intake results in hypercalcemia, and granulomatous diseases (sarcoidosis or tuberculosis). Other causes include thyrotoxicosis, pheochromocytoma, and medications such as thiazide diuretics

Table 10.1 Causes of hypercalcemia

PTH dependent
Primary hyperparathyroidism
Adenoma
Hyperplasia
Inherited syndromes – MEN and hyperparathyroidism-jaw tumor syndrome
Parathyroid carcinoma
Familial hypocalciuric hypercalcemia (FHH)
Non-PTH dependent
Hypercalcemia of malignancy
Paraneoplastic syndrome (PTHrP)
Osteolytic metastases (IL-1)
Excess 1,25 D production
Milk-alkali (calcium-alkali) syndrome
Vitamin D or A toxicity
Granulomatous diseases (sarcoidosis, tuberculosis, fungal infections)
Hormonal disorders (hyperthyroidism, acromegaly, pheochromocytoma, adrenal insufficiency)
Medications (thiazide diuretics, lithium)
Prolonged immobilization, parenteral nutrition

and lithium. In general, severe hypercalcemia is almost always a result of hyperparathyroidism or malignancy.

Presentation

The majority of patients with hypercalcemia are asymptomatic. In general, symptoms of hypercalcemia usually present when the calcium level is >12 mg/dL. The presence and severity of symptoms may be related to the time course of the rise in calcium level. If the hypercalcemia is chronic, patients may have nonspecific and relatively well-tolerated symptoms such as fatigue, constipation, and depression. A more acute rise in the calcium level to the 12–14 mg/dL range will likely result in more noticeable symptoms such as muscle weakness, nausea, abdominal pain, polyuria/

polydipsia, irritability, and changes in sensorium. Calcium levels of >13 mg/dL may result in cardiovascular complications noted on an electrocardiogram as a prolonged PR interval and a shortened QT interval, a result of a shortened myocardial action potential. Arrhythmias have been reported in patients with severe hypercalcemia.

Diagnostic Approach

The most important initial step in the evaluation of severe hypercalcemia is repeating and confirming the laboratory test result and correcting the calcium level for the albumin to obtain an accurate calcium result (Table 10.2). This correction is done using the following formula: corrected calcium (mg/dL) = measured total Ca (mg/dL) + 0.8 (4.0 − serum albumin [g/dL]), where 4.0 represents the average albumin level. If the patient has prior calcium levels recorded, these should be reviewed to determine time course of the hypercalcemia. The level and chronicity of calcium elevation can be helpful in determining the cause of hypercalcemia. Patients with primary hyperparathyroidism usually have milder and more chronic calcium elevations, compared with patients with hypercalcemia of malignancy.

Once the level of hypercalcemia has been confirmed, an intact PTH level should be measured. This will then guide further workup and management. An elevated or high/normal PTH level is consistent with a diagnosis of primary hyperparathyroidism. Although the majority of patients with this diagnosis will have a PTH well above the upper limit of normal, some patients with primary hyperparathyroidism will have an intact PTH level in the normal range. If the level is in the high/normal range, then primary hyperparathyroidism is still the most likely diagnosis, as the

Table 10.2 Initial evaluation of patients with severe hypercalcemia

1. Repeat calcium level and correct for albumin
2. Serum PTH level to distinguish PTH-mediated versus non-PTH-mediated hypercalcemia

PTH should be suppressed in patients with an elevated calcium level for causes other than hyperparathyroidism. The PTH should be low in cases of non-PTH-dependent hypercalcemia.

Most patients with PTH-dependent hypercalcemia have mild calcium elevations. There are circumstances, however, where PTH-dependent hypercalcemia can be more severe. If the patient has severe hypercalcemia and an elevated PTH, then the diagnosis of parathyroid carcinoma or a large parathyroid adenoma should be considered. These patients often have much higher PTH levels than most patients with primary hyperparathyroidism. The degree of hypercalcemia often, but not always, correlates with the PTH level. In turn, the size of the lesion can correlate with the PTH level. Patients with larger parathyroid tumors, benign or malignant, are more likely to have higher PTH levels and therefore be at higher risk for episodes of severe hypercalcemia. In patients with renal insufficiency, hypercalcemia can increase the severity because of decreased renal filtration of serum calcium.

Severe hypercalcemia is most common among patients with a non-PTH-dependent mechanism, often malignancy. In these cases, the patient frequently has more advanced malignant disease, and the diagnosis and cause of hypercalcemia may be quite obvious.

Treatment

The treatment of hypercalcemia depends primarily on the calcium level. Patients with mildly elevated levels (Ca < 12 mg/dL) often do not need treatment but should be instructed regarding factors that can exacerbate the hypercalcemia. These factors include dehydration/volume depletion, medications (thiazide diuretics and lithium therapy), prolonged bed rest or inactivity, and a high calcium diet (>1000 mg/day). It is important to instruct patients to maintain adequate hydration (at least six to eight glasses of water per day) and to consider contacting their physician if they are unable to maintain oral hydration due to illness.

The treatment of moderate hypercalcemia (12–13 mg/dL) depends on the time course of the calcium elevation and if the patient is experiencing symptoms. All patients who are acutely symptomatic should be admitted to the hospital and treated. If the calcium level is <13 mg/dL and the patient is not symptomatic, they do not necessarily require immediate treatment, but the cause of the hypercalcemia should be investigated and promptly treated to avoid further elevation in the calcium level. These patients should be instructed as outlined above regarding factors that could exacerbate the hypercalcemia and their calcium levels closely followed until the underlying cause is treated.

Any patient who has symptomatic hypercalcemia or a calcium level of >13 mg/dL should be admitted to the hospital and treatment initiated to lower the calcium level. There are four available treatment approaches to lower the calcium levels:

1. Intravenous hydration to promote excretion of calcium
2. Calcitonin
3. Bisphosphonates
4. Denosumab

The combination of intravenous hydration and calcitonin should lower calcium levels within hours, while the bisphosphonates are effective within days. The intravenous hydration to expand intravascular volume and promote calcium excretion should be initiated first. The patient's volume status should be closely assessed and monitored. The recommended infusion should start at 0.9% saline at twice the maintenance rate and the urine output monitored. The infusion rate can then be adjusted depending on the patient's age, overall medical conditions, urine output, and calcium level. It is important to expand the intravascular volume before a diuretic such as furosemide is given.

Salmon calcitonin is used in the acute setting for the treatment of hypercalcemia. It is usually administered intramuscularly or subcutaneously. The recommended starting dose is 4 international units/kg every 12 h; this can be increased up to 6–8 international units/kg every 6 h as needed. Prior to giving calcitonin, a skin test should be done to rule out any allergy to the medication.

Bisphosphonates are most effective in treating patients with malignancy-associated hypercalcemia. Bisphosphonates such as pamidronate and zoledronate inhibit osteoclast activity and therefore decrease the release of calcium from the bone. These agents are long-acting and should be used judiciously in patients with PTH-dependent hypercalcemia, as a curative operation may lead to hypocalcemia if the source of excess PTH is successfully removed and the bisphosphonates are still active in the patient's system.

Bisphosphonates should never be given to patients with hypoparathyroidism who develop iatrogenic hypercalcemia from overtreatment with calcium and vitamin D supplements. Since they lack parathyroid hormone, these patients are at risk for profound and persistent hypocalcemia with bisphosphonates. In addition, patients with renal failure should be given these agents cautiously and at a lower dose.

Denosumab can be used when bisphosphonates are contraindicated (e.g. severe renal failure). As the serum calcium level is lowered into the normal range, the cause of the hypercalcemia should be investigated and treated when possible. In the case of surgically correctable primary hyperparathyroidism, surgery should be performed as soon as possible to avoid repeated episodes of severe hypercalcemia.

An alternative for patients with hypercalcemia secondary to hyperparathyroidism is the relatively newer agent, cinacalcet. This is often an effective treatment in patients with an adenoma who are poor surgical candidates as well as for patients with inoperable parathyroid carcinoma. Once diagnosis is clarified, which will require further investigation, steroids are a therapeutic option for granulomatous disease and lymphoma mediated by 1,25-hydroxy-vitamin D production. It is also important to rule-out tuberculosis prior to administering steroids.

Summary

The most common causes of hypercalcemia in general are hyperparathyroidism and malignancy. Severe hypercalcemia can result in either of these clinical circumstances, although the majority of patients with hyperparathyroidism have mild calcium elevations. Patients with calcium levels >13 mg/dL and any patient with symptomatic hypercalcemia should be admitted to the hospital and promptly treated, with the underlying cause addressed and corrected when possible to avoid future episodes of clinically significant hypercalcemia.

Suggested Reading

Bilezikian JP, Cusano NE, Khan AA, Liu JM, Marcocci C, Bandeira F. Primary hyperparathyroidism. Nat Rev Dis Primers. 2016;2:16033.

Mohammad KS, Guise TA. Hypercalcemia of malignancy: a new twist on an old problem. J Oncol Pract. 2016;12(5):435–6.

Peacock M, Belzikian J. Cinacalcet HCL reduces hyperalcemia in primary hyperparathyroidism across a wide spectrum of disease severity. J Clin Endocrinol Metabol. 2011;96(1):E9–E18.

Srividya N, Gossman WG. Hypercalcemia. StatPearls https://knowledge.statpearls.com/chapter/acls/23158/.

Wisneski L. Salmon calcitonin in the acute management of hypercalcemia. Calcif Tissue Int. 1990;46(Suppl):S26–30.

Hypocalcemia

11

Alan Ona Malabanan

Contents

A. O. Malabanan (✉)
Beth Israel Deaconess Medical Center, Harvard Medical School,
Division of Endocrinology, Diabetes and Metabolism,
Boston, MA, USA
e-mail: amalaban@bidmc.harvard.edu

© Springer Nature Switzerland AG 2020
R. K. Garg et al. (eds.), *Handbook of Inpatient Endocrinology*,
https://doi.org/10.1007/978-3-030-38976-5_11

Hypocalcemia Should Be Considered in Those with Muscle Cramping or Bone Pain, Cardiac Dysrhythmias, Seizure Disorders, and Perioral/ Digital Paresthesias

Calcium is important for the proper functioning of several of the human body's organ systems and cellular processes. As a divalent cation, it is important in maintaining an electrochemical gradient.

Hypocalcemia is associated with tetany and muscle cramping. Latent tetany may be identified by eliciting Chvostek's or Trousseau's signs. Neurologic irritability, with hypocalcemia, is associated with oral and digital paresthesias as well as seizures. Hypocalcemia results in cardiovascular irritability with atrial and ventricular dysrhythmias and may also cause laryngospasm with respiratory arrest. Calcium is important, along with phosphate, for normal bone mineralization. Inadequate serum calcium will lead to osteomalacia and bone pain.

A Total Serum Calcium Should Be Measured with a Concomitant Serum Albumin

The most commonly measured serum calcium level is total serum calcium. About half of the total serum calcium is bound to albumin or complexed with organic ions such as phosphate. The calcium unbound to albumin or complexed with organic ions is termed the free calcium, which is the physiologically important portion. Free calcium levels are therefore affected by albumin levels. Hypoalbuminemia will lead to a decrease in total serum calcium levels. If the albumin is less than 4.0 g/dl, the total serum calcium should be corrected by adding 0.8 mg/dl of calcium to every 1.0 g/dl of albumin below 4.0.

A Free Ionized Serum Calcium from Venous Blood Gas Testing May Provide a Timelier Test Result than Total Serum Calcium

A total serum calcium level may take hours to return, while a free ionized serum calcium from an arterial blood gas analyzer often takes minutes to return, related to the assay methodology used. For patients with rapidly declining calcium levels, a free ionized serum calcium from venous blood gas testing may have an advantage in being able to adjust therapy. Accurate ionized calcium results require proper specimen collection and timely processing.

The Free Serum Calcium Decreases with Alkalemia and Increases with Acidemia

Acid-base balance affects the negative charges on albumin. Acidemia (i.e., increased H+ ions) decreases them leading to decreased ionized calcium binding to albumin and increasing free calcium. Alkalemia (i.e., decreased H+ ions) increases them leading to increased ionized calcium binding and decreasing free calcium. Respiratory alkalemia from hyperventilation will lower free calcium levels and may precipitate tetany or seizures.

The Electrocardiographic QT Interval Is Prolonged in Those with Hypocalcemia

The presence of QT prolongation confirms the risk of cardiovascular sequelae of hypocalcemia and should prompt urgent evaluation and treatment. Since electrocardiographic assessment may produce a result even more quickly than a venous blood gas, this is the quickest way for assessing calcium status in a patient.

Post-parathyroidectomy and Post-thyroidectomy Patients Should Be Monitored Postoperatively for Symptoms and Physical Signs of Hypocalcemia, as Well as an Estimate of Free Calcium

The risk of hypocalcemia after thyroid or parathyroid surgery is dependent on the type of surgery performed as well as the skill and experience of the surgeon. Preoperative vitamin D deficiency may also increase the risk for postoperative hypocalcemia. Four gland exploration/subtotal parathyroidectomy and total thyroidectomy for thyroid cancer or Graves' disease have an increased risk for hypocalcemia. Hungry bone syndrome post-parathyroidectomy is increased in those with severe primary or secondary hyperparathyroidism associated with lower bone density and increased bone turnover. Prophylactic treatment with calcium and calcitriol, as well as correction of preexisting vitamin D deficiency, may reduce the risk for symptomatic hypocalcemia post-thyroidectomy. Postoperative calcium and parathyroid hormone may be helpful in guiding postoperative management. Assessment for a baseline Chvostek's sign should be done before surgery as 10% of normal individuals may have a Chvostek's sign.

Hypocalcemia Should Be Evaluated with an Estimate of Free Serum Calcium (Free Ionized Calcium or Total Serum Calcium Corrected for Serum Albumin), Serum Phosphate, Serum Magnesium, Serum 25-Hydroxyvitamin D, and Serum Parathyroid Hormone (PTH)

Once a low free calcium is confirmed, the laboratory evaluation of hypocalcemia can suggest its etiology and need for additional supportive treatment beyond calcium. PTH is responsible for increasing calcium release from bone to normalize serum calcium levels. At the same time, increased PTH causes phosphaturia and leads to hypophosphatemia. Ineffective PTH action may result from hypomagnesemia, and hypomagnesemia may also impair PTH release. Severe vitamin D deficiency, especially if long-standing with depletion of bone calcium stores, may cause hypocalcemia. Hungry bone syndrome is characterized by low calcium, phosphate, and magnesium resulting from the reincorporation of these bone mineral components after cure of the hyperparathyroidism.

Symptomatic Hypocalcemia Is a Medical Emergency, Particularly When Acute and Should Be Treated with Intravenous 10% Calcium Gluconate (with EKG Monitoring) Until the Symptoms Resolve

Seizures, tetany, cardiac dysrhythmias, paresthesias, laryngospasm/stridor, or prolonged QT interval should be treated urgently with intravenous calcium gluconate (with EKG monitoring). Calcium gluconate is used in preference to calcium chloride, due to calcium chloride's vein irritation. One to two amps (10–20 mL) of 10% calcium gluconate may be infused over 10 min watching for bradycardia. Those with chronic kidney disease or on concomitant digoxin therapy should be infused more cautiously.

After Emergent Treatment with Intravenous Calcium Gluconate, a Calcium Gluconate IV Drip Should Be Maintained (with EKG Monitoring) Titrating the Free Serum Calcium Estimate to the Lower Limit of Normal

Because free calcium is rapidly filtered into the glomerulus, serum calcium levels will drop without an ongoing source of calcium, and hypocalcemia will recur. With EKG monitoring, a calcium gluconate IV drip using 100 ml of 10% calcium gluconate in 1 L of D5W may be started at 30 ml/h titrating to symptoms, free calcium levels, or QT intervals. Free calcium levels should be monitored every 2–4 h.

Chronic Treatment of Hypocalcemia Includes Treating the Underlying Causes (Hypomagnesemia, Vitamin D Deficiency, Inadequate Calcium Intake, Hypoparathyroidism, Hypercalciuria) and, in Addition, May Include 500–1000 mg of Elemental Calcium (1250–2500 mg of Calcium Carbonate) tid Along with an Activated Vitamin D Analog Such as Calcitriol (0.25–0.50 mcg bid)

Underlying causes of hypocalcemia, such as hypomagnesemia, vitamin D deficiency, hypercalciuria due to loop diuretics, or use of potent antiresorptives such as bisphosphonates or denosumab, should be addressed. Hypomagnesemia may require intravenous treatment with magnesium sulfate (see *Hypomagnesemia*). Vitamin D deficiency can be treated with high-dose ergocalciferol (50,000 IU weekly × 8 weeks) followed by 2000 IU cholecalciferol daily, although those with gastric bypass surgery or intestinal malabsorption may require higher doses of 6000–10,000 IU daily. Bisphosphonates should be discontinued until the hypocalcemia is corrected, and dose reduction or cessation of loop diuretics should be considered (Table 11.1).

Serum Calcium, Albumin, Phosphate, Creatinine, and 24-h Urine Calcium and Creatinine Should Be Monitored Closely and Therapy Adjusted Accordingly

The target free calcium should be in the low normal range. The calcium-phosphate product should be maintained <55 mg^2/dl^2 to minimize the risk for soft tissue calcification. The 24-h urine calcium excretion should be maintained <250 mg/day to minimize the risk for nephrolithiasis.

Thiazide Therapy Should Be Used with Extreme Caution in Those Also on Calcium and Calcitriol, Particularly if There Is Concomitant Chronic Kidney Disease

Thiazides decrease urinary calcium excretion and together with calcium and calcitriol therapy may cause hypercalcemia. Because thiazides decrease urinary excretion of calcium, the hypercalcemia is more difficult to treat.

Potent Antiresorptive Therapy with Oral and Intravenous Bisphosphonates or Subcutaneous Denosumab Is Contraindicated in Those with Hypocalcemia

Bisphosphonates and denosumab inhibit osteoclast-mediated bone resorption and prevent calcium release from the bone, disrupting calcium homeostasis and causing hypocalcemia. As such,

Table 11.1 Medications used for hypocalcemia

Medication	Mechanism of action	Route of administration	Dose (elemental calcium)	Comments
Calcium carbonate	Source of calcium	Oral	1250–2500 mg tid (500–1000 mg tid)	Requires gastric acid to aid dissolution and absorption
Calcium citrate	Source of calcium	Oral	2992–4488 mg tid (630–945 mg tid)	Oral preparation of choice in those with achlorhydria
Calcium acetate	Source of calcium	Oral	2001–4002 mg tid (507–1014 mg tid)	Typically used as a phosphate binder
Calcium gluconate (1000 mg/10 mL)	Source of calcium	Intravenous	1000–2000 mg for symptomatic hypocalcemia (93–186 mg) then 30 mL/h of 100 mL in 1 L D5W as infusion titrating to calcium.	
Calcium chloride (1000 mg/10 mL)	Source of calcium	Intravenous	500–1000 mg for symptomatic hypocalcemia (136–273 mg)	Give only as slow IV injection due to vein sclerosis
Ergocalciferol (50,000 IU)	Vitamin D2	Oral	50,000–100,000 daily to weekly	Fat soluble and long half-life, by prescription only
Cholecalciferol	Vitamin D3	Oral	50,000–100,000 daily to weekly	Fat soluble and long half-life, OTC
Calcitriol	Activated vitamin D	Oral, IV	0.25–0.50 mcg twice daily	Onset of action in 1–2 days

Hydrochlorothiazide	Hypocalciuric thiazide	Oral	25–50 mg twice daily	Hyperuricemia, hypokalemia, and hyponatremia may result
Chlorthalidone	Hypocalciuric thiazide	Oral	25–50 mg once daily	Hyperuricemia, hypokalemia, and hyponatremia may result
Amiloride	Mild hypocalciuric diuretic	Oral	5–10 mg once daily	Potassium-sparing diuretic; may be used in combination with thiazides
Parathyroid hormone (1–84)	PTH	Subcutaneous	50–100 mcg once daily	REMS necessary to prescribe, osteosarcoma risk

they are contraindicated in those patients with hypocalcemia or known hypoparathyroidism.

Long-Term Parathyroid Hormone (1–84 PTH Analog) Is Now Approved by the FDA for the Management of Chronic Hypoparathyroidism

Replacement therapy with once daily 80 mcg parathyroid hormone is now available and can decrease oral calcium and calcitriol requirements. However, its role in inpatient management of hypocalcemia is not yet clear. Long-term safety is also unclear.

Suggested Reading

Cooper MS, Gittoes NJL. Diagnosis and management of hypocalcaemia. BMJ. 2008;336:1298–302. https://doi.org/10.1136/bmj.39582.589433.BE.

Mannstadt M, Bilezikian JP, Thakker RV, Hannan FM, Clarke BL, Rejnmark L, et al. Hypoparathyroidism. Nat Rev Dis Primers. 2017;3:17055. https://doi.org/10.1038/nrdp.2017.55.

Mathur A, Nagarajan N, Kahan S, Schneider EB, Zeiger MA. Association of parathyroid hormone level with postthyroidectomy hypocalcemia: a systematic review. JAMA Surg. 2018;153:69–76. https://doi.org/10.1001/jamasurg.2017.3398.

Ross DS, Burch HB, Cooper DS, Greenlee MC, Laurberg P, Maia AL, et al. 2016 American Thyroid Association guidelines for diagnosis and management of hyperthyroidism and other causes of thyrotoxicosis. Thyroid. 2016;26:1343–421. https://doi.org/10.1089/thy.2016.0229.

Witteveen JE, van Thiel S, Romijn JA, Hamdy NA. Therapy of endocrine disease: hungry bone syndrome: still a challenge in the post-operative management of primary hyperparathyroidism: a systematic review of the literature. Eur J Endocrinol. 2013;168:R45–53. https://doi.org/10.1530/EJE-12-0528.

Perioperative Evaluation of Primary Hyperparathyroidism

12

J. Carl Pallais

Contents

J. C. Pallais (✉)
Brigham and Women's Hospital, Division of Endocrinology,
Department of Medicine, Boston, MA, USA
e-mail: jpallais@bwh.harvard.edu

© Springer Nature Switzerland AG 2020
R. K. Garg et al. (eds.), *Handbook of Inpatient Endocrinology*,
https://doi.org/10.1007/978-3-030-38976-5_12

Confirm the Preoperative Diagnosis of Primary Hyperparathyroidism

Primary hyperparathyroidism is confirmed by the findings of inappropriately elevated parathyroid hormone (PTH) levels in the setting of hypercalcemia without renal failure. PTH-dependent hypercalcemia in the setting of prolonged renal failure could indicate tertiary hyperparathyroidism. Calcium levels should be corrected for serum albumin. Occasionally the PTH levels will be within the normal range despite hypercalcemia. Because elevated calcium levels normally suppress PTH secretion, "normal" PTH levels in the setting of hypercalcemia indicate inappropriately increased PTH secretion.

In patients in whom previously normal calcium levels cannot be confirmed, measurement of 24-hour urine calcium is important to differentiate primary hyperparathyroidism from familial hypocalciuric hypercalcemia (FHH). The latter condition is a contraindication for parathyroidectomy as it is associated with a high risk of surgical failure. In these patients, hypercalcemia typically recurs with subtotal parathyroidectomy.

Review the Indications for Parathyroidectomy

Parathyroidectomy is indicated for patients with primary hyperparathyroidism and symptomatic kidney stones or fragility fractures. According to the recent guidelines, asymptomatic patients with primary hyperparathyroidism should be considered candidates for parathyroidectomy if they have any of the following indications:

- Age <50 years old
- Calcium levels >1 mg/dL above the upper limits of normal
- Abnormal renal function
- Osteoporosis at any site (spine, hip, or distal wrist)
- Presence of vertebral fracture on dedicated imaging studies
- Presence of kidney stones on abdominal imaging
- High risk of developing kidney stones on 24-hour urine analysis

Some patients may require urgent parathyroidectomy if they develop hypercalcemic crisis. This is characterized by the rapid onset of hypercalcemia, usually with calcium levels greater than 14 mg/dL, and evidence of multiorgan dysfunction. Aggressive fluid resuscitation and medical management are required prior to parathyroidectomy.

Parathyroidectomy can also be considered in patients with primary hyperparathyroidism without any of these indications if there are barriers to long-term follow-up. Surgical intervention is the only definitive treatment for primary hyperparathyroidism and could obviate the need for long-term monitoring.

Finally, parathyroidectomy can be considered in patients with primary hyperparathyroidism and no other indication if they are undergoing neck surgery for other reasons. Frequently this involves surgical evaluation of concurrent thyroid nodules. It is important to evaluate thyroid nodules in patients with primary hyperparathyroidism as the FNA results can impact the decision to undergo surgery or modify the surgical approach to parathyroidectomy.

Review Preoperative Parathyroid Imaging Studies

Imaging studies are not part of the diagnostic plan for primary hyperparathyroidism, but they help the surgeon define the surgical strategy. The most commonly utilized localizing studies are cervical ultrasounds, sestamibi parathyroid scans, and four-dimensional computed tomography (4D CT) scan. Cervical ultrasounds are relatively inexpensive, do not involve radiation exposure, and have the added benefit of detecting concomitant thyroid nodules that may impact the surgical strategy for parathyroidectomy. In 4D CT, multiple scans are obtained after administration of IV contrast and provide good anatomic detail for planning the surgery. It is important to remember that patients with negative imaging studies remain candidates for parathyroidectomy, particularly as the sensitivity of these tests are significantly lower in patients with multigland involvement.

Review the Surgical Approach

Parathyroidectomy is carried out via bilateral neck exploration or a minimally invasive approach. The choice between these two surgical strategies is determined in large part by the results of the imaging studies and the experience of the surgeon.

Bilateral parathyroid exploration has been the standard surgical approach for parathyroidectomy with a high surgical success rate of >95%. This is the preferred approach for patients with multigland disease and those with discordant or non-localizing imaging studies. Approximately 85% of cases of primary hyperparathyroidism are caused by a single adenoma. If a single adenoma is confirmed on localization studies, a focused minimally invasive operative strategy with measurement of intraoperative PTH could be attempted. PTH has a short half-life, and intraoperative monitoring helps to confirm resection of the culprit adenoma while limiting the scope of dissection. Elevated intraoperative PTH values help to identify persistent disease.

If multigland disease is discovered during surgery or an abnormal gland is not identified through a minimally invasive approach, then the surgery should be converted to bilateral exploration. Likewise, if intraoperative PTH levels do not drop appropriately after resection of an abnormal gland, conversion to bilateral exploration is recommended to avoid persistence of hyperparathyroidism. Unilateral parathyroidectomy has been associated with similar success rates as bilateral exploration in properly selected patients.

Autotransplantation of normal parathyroid glands is occasionally attempted to preserve the function of glands that appear devascularized after surgical manipulation or in subtotal parathyroidectomy with multigland involvement.

Determine Possible Association with Hereditary Syndromes

Approximately 5–10% of patients with hyperparathyroidism have an underlying hereditary syndrome, some of which are caused by mutations in known genes. These genetic syndromes∗ and their associated genes are listed below: *MEN, multiple endocrine neoplasia syndrome; HPT-JT, hyperparathyroidism-jaw tumor syndrome; and FHH, familial hypocalciuric hypercalcemia.

- MEN1 (*MEN1*)
- MEN2A (*RET*)
- MEN4 (*CDKN1B*)
- HPT-JT (HRPT2/CDC73)
- Familial isolated hyperparathyroidism
- FHH1 (*CASR*)
- FHH2 (*GNA11*)
- FHH3 (*AP2S1*)

Identification of these syndromes should ideally be done preoperatively as the diagnosis may influence the surgical strategy and may prompt screening for other associated features. Patients with hereditary syndromes associated with hyperparathyroidism tend to be younger, have multiple gland involvement, and have a greater likelihood of negative localization studies and hyperparathyroidism persistence or recurrence. Thus, screening for these syndromes should be considered in young patients with hyperparathyroidism, those with an affected first-degree relative, or patients that have other associated syndromic features. In addition, patients of any age should be considered candidates for genetic screening if they present in with multigland parathyroid disease or persistent/recurrent hyperparathyroidism following parathyroidectomy. Although parathyroidectomy is generally contraindicated for patients with FHH, the diagnosis may have been missed prior to parathyroidectomy if hypocalciuria was not identified or tested. Hypercalcemia typically persists/recurs after subtotal parathyroidectomy. These patients should not undergo repeat parathyroid operations.

Obtain Biochemical Evidence of Surgical Cure

The immediate goal of parathyroidectomy in patients with primary hyperparathyroidism is to reestablish normal calcium homeostasis. Persistent disease is manifested as a failure to achieve normocalcemia within 6 months of surgery. Operative failure may be predicted by inadequate decrease in intraoperative PTH levels. If normocalcemia is achieved for at least 6 months following parathyroidectomy, patients are considered to have had a surgical cure. Primary hyperparathyroidism that recurs after 6 months of normocalcemia following parathyroidectomy is considered recurrent disease.

Monitor for Postoperative Hypocalcemia

Postoperative hypocalcemia is the most common endocrine complication following parathyroidectomy, occurring in nearly 50% of cases in some case series. Injury to the parathyroid glands, inadvertent resection of parathyroid tissue, damaged blood supply to the remaining parathyroid glands, or failed auto-transplantation can cause transient or permanent hypoparathy-roidism. In addition to functional hypoparathyroidism, the reversal of bone resorption with increased bone formation after parathyroidectomy causes a net influx of calcium into bones contributing to the fall of serum calcium levels. Typically, the hypocalcemia is transient because the bone disease is mild and the remaining parathyroid tissue recovers function within 1 or 2 weeks. In the hands of high-volume parathyroid surgeons, permanent hypoparathyroidism is relatively uncommon after initial parathyroid surgery with an estimated frequency of <4%. Severe hypocalcemia caused by hungry bone is a rare complication of parathyroidectomy.

Hypocalcemia may be symptomatic or asymptomatic and may be associated with variable PTH levels. The duration and severity of hypocalcemia vary and may depend on the routine use of calcium and vitamin D supplementation, the degree of injury to the remaining parathyroid glands, the severity of the underlying bone disease, and preoperative clinical features. Patients with impaired intestinal absorption such as those with prior gastric bypass surgery, vitamin D deficiency, renal dys-function, or hypomagnesemia are at higher risk of developing postoperative hypocalcemia.

Evaluate for Signs and Symptoms of Postsurgical Hypocalcemia

Acute hypocalcemia may be associated with a spectrum of clinical manifestations. At the mild end of the spectrum, asymptomatic biochemical findings may be the only manifestations. Severe findings include laryngospasm, neurocognitive dysfunction, papilledema, seizures, and heart failure. Neuromuscular irritability is the most common manifestation of acute hypocalcemia. This includes perioral numbness, acral paresthesias, muscle cramps, stiffness, or carpopedal spasms. On physical exam, patients may have Chvostek's signs and/or Trousseau's sign, which are markers of latent tetany. Chvostek's sign is the contraction of the facial muscles in response to tapping the facial nerve which causes twitching of the ipsilateral lip. Trousseau's sign is the development of carpal spam characterized by adduction of the thumb, extension of the interphalangeal joints, and flexion of the MCP joints and wrist elicited by the insufflation of a blood pressure cuff above the systolic blood pressure for 3 min. Trousseau's sign is more specific for hypocalcemia as Chvostek's sign may be present in up to 10% of normal subjects. Hypocalcemia may also cause QTc prolongation and may be associated with dysrhythmias.

Evaluate for Biochemical Evidence of Hypoparathyroidism

The biochemical signature of hypoparathyroidism involves hypocalcemia with suppressed PTH levels. Approximately 40% of the total circulating calcium is bound to albumin, with the unbound or free portion referred to as ionized calcium. Total calcium measurement should be corrected for albumin levels according to the following formula: corrected calcium (mg/dL) = measured calcium (mg/dL) + 0.8 (4.0 – measured albumin [g/dL]).

If hypocalcemia is confirmed by either corrected calcium measurement or ionized calcium levels, hypoparathyroidism is diagnosed if the PTH levels are inappropriately suppressed.

As hypocalcemia normally elevates PTH levels, PTH values within the normal range are still considered inappropriately low in the setting of hypocalcemia.

PTH increases circulating calcium levels by stimulating calcium efflux from the bone, promoting reabsorption of filtered calcium in the kidney, and indirectly increasing intestinal calcium absorption by promoting the activation of vitamin D through the expression of 1-alpha hydroxylase in the proximal tubule. Suppressed PTH release due to the resection or injury of parathyroid glands lowers serum calcium levels by reversing these physiologic processes. In addition, PTH is one of the primary regulators of phosphorus in the body and promotes urinary phosphate excretion thorough its effects on the NaPi transporters in the proximal tubules. In hypoparathyroidism, the serum phosphorous concentration tends to be in the high-normal or frankly elevated range due to impaired phosphate excretion.

As low magnesium levels can impair PTH secretion and action, it is important to exclude hypomagnesemia as the cause of hypoparathyroidism or as a contributor to the hypocalcemia.

Assess for Evidence of the Hungry Bone Syndrome

Patients with severe preoperative bone disease caused by chronic bone resorption mediated by elevated PTH levels may have severe and prolonged hypocalcemia following parathyroidectomy. The reversal of advanced bone resorption from the acute withdrawal of PTH is coupled with accelerated bone formation and causes a strong influx of both calcium and phosphate into the bone in these patients. This lowers the calcium levels despite a compensatory increase in PTH production by the remaining parathyroid tissue.

The clinical markers of the hungry bone syndrome include persistent hypocalcemia and hypophosphatemia on postoperative day 3 following parathyroidectomy. The hypocalcemia typically nadirs 2–4 days after parathyroidectomy but may last up to several months. In addition to low serum phosphorous concentrations, associated biochemical features frequently include hypomagnesemia and occasionally hyperkalemia. Risk factors for developing the hungry bone syndrome include large volume of the resected adenoma, elevated preoperative blood urea nitrogen level, elevated preoperative alkaline phosphatase activity, older age, and preoperative radiographic findings of osteitis fibrosa or bone erosions. Occasionally, patients with bone disease caused by hyperthyroidism may also develop the hungry bone syndrome following thyroidectomy. This must be a consideration for patients undergoing combined thyroid and parathyroid surgeries.

Prevent and Treat Hypocalcemia

Regular monitoring of calcium, albumin, phosphorus, magnesium, and vitamin D levels and occasional PTH measurements are required after parathyroidectomy to confirm surgical cure and detect development of hypocalcemia. Oral calcium and vitamin D supplementation are commonly started immediately following parathyroidectomy to prevent hypocalcemia. Between 1.5 and 3 g of elemental calcium is typically given orally in divided doses in the postoperative periods for several days to weeks depending on the serum calcium and PTH concentrations. Aggressive vitamin D repletion with high-dose ergocalciferol or cholecalciferol can be considered in patients with preoperative vitamin D deficiency.

Most cases of hypocalcemia are mild and can be treated with oral calcium and vitamin D supplementation in the outpatient setting. As the hypocalcemia worsens, the dose of elemental calcium is increased. For patients with achlorhydria or on proton pump inhibitors, the use of the calcium citrate formulation is preferred over calcium carbonate for improved calcium absorption. For symptomatic patients or those who have developed hypoparathyroidism, calcitriol may be added to their regimen. Calcitriol is the bioactive form of vitamin D, has a faster onset of action than ergocalciferol or cholecalciferol, and is more effective in stimulating intestinal calcium absorption. However, because of its greater potency, it has a narrower therapeutic window, and careful monitoring is required to ensure that serum or urinary calcium levels do not become excessively elevated.

Patients with more severe hypocalcemia may require longer hospital stays as their hypocalcemia may represent a medical emergency. Intravenous calcium administration should be considered for patients with moderate to severe symptoms of hypocalcemia or those with corrected calcium levels <7.5 mg/dL or ionized calcium concentrations <1.0 mmol/L. The typical starting dose is 1–2 g of IV calcium gluconate administered over 10–20 min. This bolus dose translates to approximately 90–180 mg of elemental calcium. Following the IV bolus, a continuous infusion of calcium gluconate of approximately 50–100 mg of elemental calcium/h can be initiated for several hours until symptoms resolve. Transition to oral calcium and calcitriol can then be initiated. In hypoparathyroidism or the hungry bone syndrome, large calcium doses may be required to facilitate enteral calcium absorption. Calcitriol doses can range from 0.25 to 4 mcg per day. As magnesium depletion may impair PTH release as well as its action, aggressive magnesium replacement is required. In contrast, phosphate administration is typically avoided in patients with hypophosphatemia and hypocalcemia as it can bind to calcium and further lower ionized calcium concentrations. In severe cases of the hungry bone syndrome with extreme hypophosphatemia, phosphate repletion may be considered but cautious administration is advised.

Follow-Up After Discharge

The discharge plan should include a timely follow-up visit for continued evaluation of calcium concentrations. An appointment should be made for the patient within 1–2 weeks following surgery to measure the calcium and PTH levels and adjust the calcium and vitamin D doses. It is important that the patient is educated about the signs and symptoms of hypercalcemia and hypocalcemia and that they are able to contact their providers if they experience suggestive symptoms in order to have laboratory levels checked. For patients with persistent or permanent hypoparathyroidism, calcium and vitamin D/calcitriol dosing is adjusted to keep calcium levels in the lower limits of normal to prevent hypercalciuria. Thiazide diuretics may be added if hypercalciuria develops. Selected patients with hypoparathyroidism may be candidates for treatment with parathyroid hormone injections.

Suggested Reading

Bilezikian JP, Brandi ML, Eastell R, Silverberg SJ, Udelsman R, Marcocci C, et al. Guidelines for the management of asymptomatic primary hyperparathyroidism: summary statement from the Fourth International Workshop. J Clin Endocrinol Metabol. 2014;99(10):3561–9.

Jain N, Reilly RF. Hungry bone disease. Curr Opin Nephrol Hypertens. 2017;26(4):250–5.

Stack BC Jr, Bimston DN, Bodenner DL, Brett EM, Dralle H, Orloff LA, et al. American association of clinical endocrinologists and American college of endocrinology disease state clinical review: postoperative hypoparathyroidism–definitions and management. Endocr Pract. 2015;21(6): 674–85.

Udelsman R, Akerstrom G, Biagini C, Duh QY, Miccoli P, Niederle B, et al. The surgical management of asymptomatic primary hyperparathyroidism: proceedings of the Fourth International Workshop. J Clin Endocrinol Metabol. 2014;99(10):3595–606.

Wilhelm SM, Wang TS, Ruan DT, Lee JA, Asa SL, Duh QY, et al. The American association of endocrine surgeons guidelines for definitive management of primary hyperparathyroidism. JAMA Surg. 2016;151(10): 959–68.

Management of Osteoporosis in the Inpatient Setting

13

Marcy A. Cheifetz

Contents

M. A. Cheifetz (✉)
Harvard Vanguard Medical Associates, Atrius Health, Department of
Endocrinology, Chestnut Hill, MA, USA
e-mail: marcy_cheifetz@atriushealth.org

© Springer Nature Switzerland AG 2020   145
R. K. Garg et al. (eds.), *Handbook of Inpatient Endocrinology*,
https://doi.org/10.1007/978-3-030-38976-5_13

Definition of Osteoporosis

Osteoporosis is defined as a disease of low bone mass and abnormal bone microarchitecture that leads to decreased bone strength and increased risk of fragility fracture. The term "fragility fracture" indicates a fracture that would not occur when bone strength and quality are normal, such as after a fall from a standing height. Osteoporotic fractures are defined as fragility fractures that occur at the vertebrae, hip, wrist, humerus, or pelvis. Although it has been well established that osteoporosis can be diagnosed with a bone density test, it is not as well appreciated that osteoporosis can also be diagnosed clinically. A hip or vertebral fragility fracture is synonymous with a clinical diagnosis of osteoporosis. Fragility fractures become increasingly prevalent as people age. Worldwide, one in three women and one in five men over age 50 will experience a fragility fracture in their lifetime. Fragility fractures that are most commonly seen in the inpatient setting include fractures of the hip and vertebrae. Hip fractures are particularly prevalent among the elderly population, especially for those residing in long-term care institutions who are most prone to imbalance and falls.

Significance of Fragility Fractures

Osteoporotic fragility fractures are associated with significant morbidity, as well as an increased risk of mortality. The osteoporotic fractures most associated with negative health outcomes are hip fractures and vertebral fractures. Hip fractures, in particular, are associated with significant morbidity and an increased risk of mortality. At 1-year post-hip fracture, mortality rates reach nearly 40% in men and 25% in women, and mortality rates have been shown to remain elevated for up to 5–15 years after the fracture. Increased mortality rates have also been seen after fragility fractures of the spine. A prior fragility fracture of the hip or vertebrae confers up to a fivefold increased risk of future fracture. For these reasons, prevention of future fracture is of the utmost importance. However less than 20% of patients admitted with fragility fractures of the hip or spine ultimately receive osteoporosis treatment.

Fragility Fractures of the Hip

The majority of patients who are admitted to the hospital with a hip fracture will require surgical intervention. Approximately 50% of hip fracture patients never regain their prior level of physical function, and many do not return to independent living. A high percentage report chronic pain even after 1-year postfracture. Approximately half of all patients who present with a hip fracture have already had a previous fragility fracture.

Fragility Fractures of the Vertebra

Vertebral fragility fractures are a common occurrence in the older osteoporosis population. Vertebral fractures also can have significant adverse effects on quality of life, and mortality rates are also substantial, with some studies showing over 20% greater age-adjusted mortality rates in women with one or more vertebral fractures. Furthermore, vertebral fractures can cause or exacerbate kyphosis, restrictive lung disease, and chronic pain. Although they may be triggered by a fall or trauma, fragility fractures of the spine can occur spontaneously without a known inciting event. Two-thirds of vertebral fragility fractures are asymptomatic. The third that are clinically symptomatic can present with severe pain and associated disability that may necessitate hospitalization. The majority of cases can be managed conservatively with institution of pain control measures and physical therapy, as tolerated. In cases where adequate pain control cannot be achieved, vertebral augmentation with either percutaneous vertebroplasty or balloon kyphoplasty may be considered. However, whether such procedures are truly effective remains controversial. Overall, management of the vertebral fracture patient often requires a multidisciplinary approach that may involve pain management, interventional radiology, neurosurgery, and physical therapy.

Inpatient Management of Fragility Fractures

There are many interventions that can be instituted by the inpatient care team for patients with fragility fractures. Non-pharmacological interventions such as initiation of calcium and vitamin D for those not already taking supplementation should be standard of care to help ensure adequate mineral stores and reduce the risk of secondary hyperparathyroidism and osteomalacia. Additionally, ensuring adequate nutritional status is vital, particularly in the elderly population that may be more at risk for malnutrition. It is also critical to identify an individual's modifiable risk factors for falling to help potentially reduce the risk of recurrent falls and fractures in the future. Risk factors associated with falling in the elderly population include arrhythmias, impaired gait and balance, impaired vision, and neurological or musculoskeletal disorders. Interventions and treatments that address these common comorbidities can have significant benefits on reducing future fracture risks. Similarly, close scrutiny of an individual's medication list is critical to help identify and potentially discontinue or change medications that may alter mental status or balance and contribute to fall risk. Involvement of physical therapy to help address a patient's risk for falling and recommend fall-prevention measures that can be instituted as an outpatient is also an important aspect of the care of these patients. The initiation of pharmacologic treatment for osteoporosis should also be considered in the inpatient setting after an acute fragility fracture (see Table 13.1). In the presence of a fragility fracture of the hip or spine, which is indicative of osteoporosis regardless of bone density status, it is not necessary to obtain a bone density test before initiating osteoporosis treatment. Osteoporosis treatment can be instituted in the acute setting immediately after a fragility fracture and does not need to be delayed until the fracture heals. Bisphosphonates, such as alendronate, risedronate, and zoledronic acid, are the most commonly utilized osteoporosis medications for osteoporosis. Studies have shown that bisphosphonates significantly reduce the risk of future fracture by 50–70% at the spine and 40–50% at the hip over 3–5 years of treatment in patients with or without prevalent vertebral fracture. The Horizon

Table 13.1 Acute fragility fracture pharmacologic therapy

Drug	Start after fracture and when	Continue after acute fracture	When to resume if stopped after acute fracture	Comment
Bisphosphonate Alendronate Risedronate Zoledronic acid	Yes. Can be initiated within 2 weeks of fracture	Yes	–	Discontinue in setting of atypical femur fracture (AFF)
Anabolic therapy Teriparatide Abaloparatide	Yes. Can be initiated within 1 week of fracture, although data limited to case reports and small clinical trials	Yes	–	Avoid in setting of preexisting hyperparathyroidism, hypercalcemia, nephrolithiasis, Paget's disease of the bone, history of skeletal malignancy, or history of radiation to skeleton
SERM Raloxifene	Not first line. Can be initiated immediately after fracture in the absence of DVT but limited by lack of efficacy in preventing non-vertebral fractures	No	Only if and when back to baseline ambulatory status as an outpatient	Associated with increased DVT risk, which may be exacerbated by immobility, and with small increased stroke risk. Discontinue in setting of DVT, MI, stroke or immobility.

(continued)

Table 13.1 (continued)

Drug	Start after fracture and when	Continue after acute fracture	When to resume if stopped after acute fracture	Comment
Anti-rank ligand Denosumab	Can be initiated immediately after fracture	Yes	–	Should be discontinued in setting of AFF. Should not be abruptly discontinued without transition to bisphosphonate due to risk of rebound vertebral fracture.
Romosozumab	Likely can be initiated immediately after fracture but data re: effects on fracture healing not yet available	Yes	–	Given association with increased CV risks, should be discontinued in setting of MI or stroke.
HRT	Not first line	No	Only if and when back to baseline ambulatory status as an outpatient	In oral forms, estrogen is associated with increased DVT risk, which may be exacerbated by immobility. Discontinue in the setting of DVT, MI, stroke, or immobility

Recurrent Fracture Trial, a randomized, controlled trial of yearly zoledronic acid administered to hip fracture patients within 90 days after surgical repair, showed a 35% relative risk reduction in rates of any new clinical fracture over the ensuing 2 years compared to placebo. Furthermore, in this same study, the group that received zoledronic acid experienced an almost 30% reduction in mortality from any cause, a particularly important finding given the known association of hip fracture with increased mortality. Additionally, there was no difference seen in the incidence of delayed union between the zoledronic acid group and the placebo group, suggesting that there is no evidence of impaired fracture healing when bisphosphonate therapy is initiated within 90 days of hip fracture repair. In a separate analysis, there was similarly no effect on healing seen with different timing intervals even when zoledronic acid was administered within 2 weeks of hip fracture repair. Other studies examining oral bisphosphonates such as alendronate and risedronate demonstrated similar findings, with no relationship seen between the use or timing of bisphosphonates on healing of femoral, humeral, or distal radius fractures even when administered within 2 weeks of the fracture event.

Prior to administration of bisphosphonate treatment, particularly intravenous zoledronic acid, vitamin D deficiency must be corrected in order to avoid development of hypocalcemia. In the aforementioned Horizon Recurrent Fracture Trial, vitamin D levels were measured prior to zoledronic acid infusion, with levels below 15 ng/mL treated with a loading dose of vitamin D 50,000–120,000 units orally or intramuscularly 2 weeks prior to the first infusion of IV zoledronic acid, followed by daily calcium 1000–1500 mg and daily vitamin D 800–1200 IU thereafter. Due to the high incidence of vitamin D deficiency found in this population, the study protocol was ultimately changed so that all enrolled patients received a loading dose of vitamin D 2 weeks prior to the initial zoledronic acid infusion regardless of baseline vitamin D levels.

In addition to vitamin D deficiency, renal dysfunction may also prove to be a limiting factor with the use of bisphosphonates, particularly in the hospital setting. Oral bisphosphonates should not be administered below an estimated creatinine clearance of

30–35 ml/min, and intravenous zoledronic acid should not be administered below an estimated creatinine clearance of 35 ml/min.

The anabolic agents teriparatide and abaloparatide have also been shown to be efficacious for the treatment of osteoporosis and osteoporotic fractures. Teriparatide, which is a recombinant form of PTH (1–34), and abaloparatide, which is an analog of PTH-related peptide (PTH-rp), both exert their anabolic effects through stimulation of the PTH receptor. The net effect of this stimulation is increased recruitment and activation of osteoblasts and enhancement of bone formation. In addition to their proven role in reducing the risk of vertebral and non-vertebral fracture, there has been growing evidence that these anabolic agents may also have beneficial effects on fracture healing. Several small studies and case reports of teriparatide have demonstrated efficacy in promoting more rapid callus formation and radiographic healing time in the acute fracture setting. Anecdotal reports have also shown positive effects of teriparatide in promoting healing in circumstances of delayed or nonunion fractures and in peri-prosthetic fractures. Furthermore, small studies have shown a possible role for teriparatide in promoting the healing of atypical femur fractures. At the present time, data for the beneficial use of abaloparatide for promoting fracture healing is limited to animal studies. Because of reports of osteosarcoma development in rats given teriparatide and abaloparatide, anabolic agents are contraindicated in individuals with a history of radiation to the skeleton, Paget's disease of the bone, bone metastases, or skeletal malignancies. Anabolic agents should also be avoided in patients with underlying hyperparathyroidism, hypercalcemia, and active nephrolithiasis. At the present time, all of the data supporting the utility of anabolic agents in the acute fracture setting come from small clinical trials or case reports, and neither of the currently available anabolic therapies have been officially approved for use in fracture repair. Larger prospective trials are needed to confirm the efficacy of anabolic therapies for the promotion of fracture healing.

Other osteoporosis agents, such as denosumab, a human monoclonal antibody against RANK-ligand, and romosozumab, a humanized monoclonal antibody to sclerostin, are not easily initiated in the inpatient setting but are similarly effective medications that could be considered as alternative choices for treatment as an outpatient.

Laboratory Evaluation

All patients with fragility fracture should undergo a comprehensive laboratory evaluation to exclude secondary causes of osteoporosis. General recommendations for screening labs include 25-hydroxyvitamin D, PTH, serum calcium, phosphate, creatinine, eGFR, and TSH. Interpretation of vitamin D levels in the inpatient setting may be confounded by the severity of the underlying illness. In the setting of critical illness, vitamin D deficiency has been found to be highly prevalent, and several meta-analyses have demonstrated an association between vitamin D deficiency and poorer outcomes. Vitamin D deficiency in the ICU population may relate to preexisting nutritional deficits or disease, but studies have shown that critical illness can also lead to dysregulation of vitamin D metabolism, further exacerbating the deficiency. In the ICU settings, this is often further compounded by fluid resuscitation, interstitial extravasation, liver dysfunction, and renal insufficiency.

In men, hypogonadism is also associated with development of osteoporosis, but testosterone should not be measured in the acute hospital setting due to an increased likelihood of falsely low levels. In cases of vertebral fracture, evaluation for multiple myeloma with measurement of serum and/or urine protein electrophoresis is also recommended. More extensive laboratory testing can be undertaken in the outpatient setting, including 24-h urine calcium measurement, to ensure calcium intake and absorption and to exclude hypercalciuria.

Continuing Pre-hospitalization Osteoporosis Medications as an Inpatient

Patients who are admitted with an acute fragility fracture and are already taking osteoporosis medication can, in most cases, continue their medication as an inpatient. As previously discussed, bisphosphonates do not significantly interfere with fracture healing and therefore can typically be continued during hospitalization for an acute fracture. However, given their long-term retention in the bone, short-term discontinuation of bisphosphonate therapy, if necessary, is unlikely to have a significant negative impact on bone health. Furthermore, bisphosphonates should not be administered in the setting of creatinine clearance below 30–35 ml/min and should be discontinued in the setting of acute renal failure. Like bisphosphonates, denosumab does not impair fracture healing or increase the risk of nonunion when administered within 6 weeks before or after a fracture, according to results from the Freedom trial. Furthermore, discontinuation of denosumab without transition to a bisphosphonate leads to significant rebound bone loss that can be associated with spontaneous vertebral fracture and therefore should be avoided in the inpatient setting. Anabolic agents such as teriparatide or abaloparatide can typically be continued in the hospitalized patient after a fragility fracture unless significant hypercalcemia is noted. In that case, the medication should be held until the hypercalcemia resolves and then can be restarted on an every other day schedule as long as there is close follow-up of calcium levels post-discharge. Raloxifene is an oral selective estrogen receptor modulator that is given daily to some postmenopausal women with osteoporosis, although it is less commonly used than other osteoporosis medications, particularly in elderly individuals, due to associated increased risk of DVT and possibly stroke. In the acute setting after hip fracture and possibly after vertebral fracture, when patients are often immobile, raloxifene should be discontinued to minimize the risk of DVT. In the absence of other contraindications, it can be restarted as an outpatient, although switching to a more potent osteoporosis agent post-discharge would be advisable, particularly since raloxifene has not been shown to reduce the risk of hip fracture. Romosozumab, a humanized monoclonal antibody to sclerostin that has been recently approved for treatment of osteoporosis for those at high risk for fracture, is administered as a subcutaneous injection once a month for up to 12 months. There is currently no data available regarding its effect on fracture healing, but given its anabolic effects it is unlikely to interfere. Since it is given monthly, administration of romosozumab in the inpatient setting would only be required during prolonged hospital stays. Romosozumab has been associated with an increased risk of cardiovascular disease, and currently the labeling includes a black box warning stating that it may increase the risk of heart attack, stroke, and cardiovascular death. If a patient experiences a heart attack or stroke during treatment, romosozumab should be discontinued.

Although osteoporosis medications can typically be continued after hospitalization for an acute fracture, one notable exception is in the case of a proven atypical femur fracture (AFF). Atypical femur fracture is a fracture of the femoral shaft that occurs after minimal or no trauma and is an extremely rare occurrence in patients receiving antiresorptive therapies, such as bisphosphonates or denosumab. The rates of AFF associated with the use of bisphosphonates in doses administered for osteoporosis treatment have been estimated at approximately 2 per 100,000 person-years after 2 years of bisphosphonate use. However, the incidence of AFF appears to increase with long-term use, with reports of 78 cases per 100,000 patient-years after 8 years of bisphosphonate exposure, most of these occurring after 5 years of use. In cases of suspected or proven AFF in a patient currently taking an oral bisphosphonate, such as alendronate, risedronate, or ibandronate, the medication should be immediately discontinued. AFFs have also been associated with denosumab use, although in the Freedom Extension Study, only one AFF was noted after 10 years of denosumab use. Similarly rare rates of AFF have been noted with romosozumab, although a causal link has not yet been definitively established. Since medications such as intravenous zoledronic acid or subcutaneous denosumab are given on a biannual or annual basis, cessation of therapy is not typically feasible in the inpatient setting, but future administration should be avoided if AFF occurs during treatment. In the case of denosumab, discontinuation leads to significant rebound bone loss and has been associated with an increased risk for spontaneous vertebral fracture; for this reason, discontinuation should be undertaken with caution and preferably with the involvement of an endocrinologist.

Preventing Future Fractures

Despite the high prevalence of osteoporotic fractures in the elderly population and the high risk of future fracture in those who have already suffered a fragility fracture, the vast majority of patients who experience such a fracture are never identified as having osteoporosis or having started on osteoporosis medication. The inpatient setting represents a unique opportunity to identify individuals as having osteoporosis and initiate interventions and anti-fracture treatment to help minimize future fracture risks. Many hospitals worldwide have instituted fracture liaison services (FLS) led by hospital-based coordinators to identify patients with fragility fracture and, using a multidisciplinary approach, facilitate bone density testing, laboratory evaluations, initiation of osteoporosis therapy, and follow-up osteoporosis care as an outpatient. Studies of FLS programs have shown significantly higher rates of treatment initiation and significantly lower rates of recurrent fracture and mortality in patients compared to patients receiving usual care.

Follow-Up After Discharge

Many patients who have suffered a fragility fracture, particularly of the hip or spine, will require physical rehabilitation after discharge, and in some cases transfer to an inpatient rehabilitation facility may be necessary. Such decisions should be made on an individualized basis. All patients who have been admitted with a fragility fracture of the hip or spine should be set up for a follow-up visit with their primary care team for further evaluation and management of their osteoporosis after discharge. A bone density test should be arranged post-discharge. If osteoporosis treatment has not been initiated during the hospitalization, patients should be discharged with instructions to follow up with their primary care doctors to initiate osteoporosis treatment as an outpatient.

Suggested Reading

Bone HG, Wagman RB, Brandi ML, Brown JP, Chapurlat R, Cummings SR, C et al. 10 years of denosumab treatment in postmenopausal women with osteoporosis: results from the phase 3 randomised FREEDOM trial and open-label extension. Lancet Diabetes Endocrinol. 2017;5(7):513–23.

Camacho PM, Petak SM, Binkley N, Clarke BL, Harris ST, Hurley DL, et al. American Association of Clinical Endocrinologists and American College of Endocrinology Clinical Practice guidelines for the diagnosis and treatment of postmenopasual osteoporosis–2016. Endocr Pract. 2016;22(9):1111–8.

Colón-Emeric C, Nordsletten L, Olson S, Major N, Boonen S, Haentjens P, HORIZON Recurrent Fracture Trial, et al. Association between timing of zoledronic acid infusion and hip fracture healing. Osteoporos Int. 2011;22(8):2329–36.

Cosman F, de Beur SJ, LeBoff MS, Lewiecki EM, Tanner B, Randall S, et al. Clinician's guide to prevention and treatment of osteoporosis. Osteoporos Int. 2014;25(10):2359–81.

Ip TP, Leung J, Kung AW. Management of osteoporosis in patients hospitalized for hip fractures. Osteoporos Int. 2010;21(Suppl 4):S605–14.

Lamy O, Gonzalez-Rodriguez E, Stoll D, Hans D, Aubry-Rozier B. Severe rebound-associated vertebral fractures after denosumab discontinuation: 9 clinical cases report. J Clin Endocrinol Metab. 2017;102(2):354–8.

Lyles KW, Colón-Emeric CS, Magaziner JS, Adachi JD, Pieper CF, Mautalen C, HORIZON Recurrent Fracture Trial, et al. Zoledronic acid and clinical fractures and mortality after hip fracture. N Engl J Med. 2007;357(18):1799–809.

Molvik H, Khan W. Bisphosphonates and their influence on fracture healing; a systematic review. Osteoporos Int. 2015;25:1251–60.

Ong T, Kantachuvesiri P, Sahota O, Gladman JRF. Characteristics and outcomes of hospitalised patients with vertebral fragility fractures: a systematic review. Age Ageing. 2018;47:17–25.

Roberts SJ, Ke HZ. Anabolic strategies to augment bone fracture healing. Curr Osteoporos Rep. 2018;16:289–98.

Sànchez-Riera L, Wilson N. Fragility fractures & their impact on older people. Best Pract Res Clin Rheumatol. 2017;31:169–91.

Wu CH, Tu ST, Chang YF, Chan DC, Chien JT, Lin CH, et al. Fracture liaison services improve outcomes of patients with osteoporosis-related fractures: a systemic literature review and meta-analysis. Bone. 2018;111: 92–100.

Calcium Disorders in End-Stage Renal Failure Including Those on Dialysis

Alan Ona Malabanan

Contents

A. O. Malabanan (✉)
Beth Israel Deaconess Medical Center, Harvard Medical School, Division of Endocrinology, Diabetes and Metabolism, Boston, MA, USA
e-mail: amalaban@bidmc.harvard.edu

© Springer Nature Switzerland AG 2020
R. K. Garg et al. (eds.), *Handbook of Inpatient Endocrinology*,
https://doi.org/10.1007/978-3-030-38976-5_14

Calcium Metabolism in Chronic Kidney Disease (CKD) Is Characterized by Aberrations in Calcium and Phosphate Clearance, Decreases in 1-α-Hydroxylase Activity with Decreased Calcium Absorption, and Parathyroid Hormone Resistance

Serum calcium is controlled by the interaction between the bone, the kidney, and the gut through the actions of dietary calcium, vitamin D, and parathyroid hormone. With the loss of kidney function, there is ultimately the loss of the 1-alpha-hydroxylase, lowering the production of 1,25-dihydroxyvitamin D and impairing gastrointestinal calcium absorption. However, aberrations in calcium metabolism occur before this critical loss of renal mass and 1-alpha-hydroxylase activity. The kidneys are also responsible for phosphate clearance, important because of the marked efficiency of gastrointestinal phosphate absorption and the omnipresence of phosphate in our diet. With increased phosphate levels, fibroblast growth factor 23 (FGF-23) increases due to its role as a phosphaturic factor. FGF-23 inhibits the renal 1-alpha-hydroxylase (since 1,25-dihydroxyvitamin D increases phosphate absorption) and lowers 1,25-dihydroxyvitamin D levels. Parathyroid hormone (PTH) rises, as compensation, increasing bone turnover and release of calcium from the bone, to maintain calcium homeostasis. In addition, hyperphosphatemia may directly stimulate PTH secretion, since PTH is also a phosphaturic factor. Worsening azotemia also results in PTH resistance, further requiring higher PTH levels to maintain calcium homeostasis.

Calcium Status in CKD Stages 3–5 Should Be Assessed with an Estimate of Ionized Calcium (i.e., Total Serum Calcium Corrected for Serum Albumin), Serum Phosphate, Serum Parathyroid Hormone, and Serum Bone-Specific Alkaline Phosphatase

Hypoalbuminemia in nephrotic syndrome may lower total serum calcium levels, so serum calcium levels should always be assessed with a concomitant serum albumin. The total serum calcium should be corrected for hypoalbuminemia (corrected serum calcium = total serum calcium + ((4.0 − Albumin) × 0.8)). Aberrations in acid-base status may necessitate a direct measurement of ionized calcium, since acidemia increases ionized calcium levels. Hyperparathyroidism is associated with bone and vascular disease and should be monitored. Appropriate ranges for PTH are typically above the normal reference range due to PTH resistance and a risk for adynamic bone disease with lower than optimal PTH levels. Bone-specific alkaline phosphatase reflects PTH action on the bone and may help in individualizing PTH targets. Optimal PTH ranges for those not on dialysis with CKD 3a to 5 are unknown. PTH has poor sensitivity and specificity in identifying high and low turnover. In addition, PTH has marked variability with regard to diet and diurnal changes. The Kidney Disease Improving Global Outcomes (KDIGO) guidelines have focused on following PTH trends rather than individual values and correcting vitamin D deficiency, hyperphosphatemia, high phosphate diet, and hypocalcemia. For those with CKD 5D, PTH target range has been recommended at 2× to 9× the upper limit of normal since high or rising PTH levels are associated with increased metabolic bone disease, morbidity, and mortality.

Calcium Disorders in CKD Should Be Managed in Close Coordination with the Patient's Primary Nephrologist, Carefully Reconciling the Medications Being Taken as an Outpatient and Being Given in Dialysis

Often patients receiving hemodialysis are followed in outpatient dialysis centers, and they have frequent lab testing as well as long-acting medications given in dialysis. It is critical to obtain these records and reconcile medication lists to plan appropriate management. Direct communication with the patient's outpatient primary nephrologist is paramount both on admission and on discharge.

Hypocalcemia Should Be Managed as Previously Described for Chronic Hypocalcemia but Being Particularly Cautious About Avoiding Hypercalcemia, an Elevated Calcium-Phosphate Product, and Parathyroid Hormone/Bone Alkaline Phosphatase Suppression

Hypocalcemia is managed by ruling out pseudo-hypocalcemia related to hypoalbuminemia and ruling out vitamin D deficiency or hypomagnesemia as a cause. Treatment is focused on correcting vitamin D deficiency, assuring adequate calcium intake and then considering activated vitamin D analogues. Because the impaired kidneys may not be able to clear excess calcium or phosphate, attention and care should be paid to avoiding hypercalcemia and an elevated calcium-phosphate product. An elevated calcium-phosphate product increases the risk for metastatic calcification of soft tissues and, as mentioned in the chapter on hypocalcemia, should be maintained <55 mg^2/dl^2.

Secondary Hyperparathyroidism May Be Managed with Dietary Phosphate Restriction or Phosphate Binding, Adequate Calcium Intake, Activated Vitamin D, or Cinacalcet Use

Hypocalcemia and hyperphosphatemia are associated with increased mortality and vascular disease, as is secondary hyperparathyroidism. The KDIGO guidelines suggest dietary phosphate restriction in the setting of hyperphosphatemia, making sure that other nutrient intake isn't compromised. Guidance and teaching from a dietitian would be helpful. It is unclear what PTH target should be considered for patients with CKD not on dialysis. KDIGO recommends PTH targets from two times upper limit of normal to nine times upper limit for those on dialysis. For those with CKD G3a-G5 and rising PTH levels, addressing modifiable etiologies such as vitamin D deficiency, hypocalcemia, and hyperphosphatemia is warranted. With hypocalcemia, calcium supplements and calcitriol, as outlined in the hypocalcemia chapter, would be indicated. If dietary phosphate restriction is insufficient to control phosphate levels, nonaluminum phosphate binders are recommended, with non-calcium phosphate binders such as sevelamer having some advantage over calcium-containing phosphate binders. Activated vitamin D therapy and calcium-based phosphate binders should not be used in patients with hypercalcemia. If serum calcium levels are high normal, paricalcitol and doxercalciferol may be preferred to calcitriol due to a lower tendency to raise serum calcium levels. Cinacalcet, a calcium sensing receptor agonist, may be helpful in lowering PTH if the above measures are unsuccessful. GI upset is a side effect. Cinacalcet should not be used in patients with hypocalcemia. Cinacalcet use might lower the incidence of mortality and cardiovascular events in older dialysis patients by lowering FGF-23 levels. Normalization of PTH and suppressing bone-specific alkaline phosphatase should be avoided to minimize the risk for adynamic bone disease.

Tertiary Hyperparathyroidism May Be Managed with Adequate Fluid Intake, Reducing Calcium and Activated Vitamin D Intake, Cinacalcet Use, or Parathyroid Surgery

Occasionally secondary hyperparathyroidism leads to worsening parathyroid hyperplasia and autonomy, eventually causing hypercalcemia, most often after renal transplantation. Maintaining adequate fluid intake and lowering or stopping the calcium and activated vitamin D may control the hypercalcemia. Cinacalcet is often started at 30 mg p.o. daily with lab testing at least 12 h after dosing. If medical therapy is insufficient to control serum calcium levels or there is significant bone involvement, surgical therapy is indicated for parathyroid debulking.

Suggested Reading

Kidney Disease: Improving Global Outcomes (KDIGO) CKD-MBD Update Work Group. KDIGO 2017 clinical practice guideline update for the diagnosis, evaluation, prevention, and treatment of chronic kidney disease–mineral and bone disorder (CKD-MBD). Kidney Int Suppl. 2017;7:1–59.

Moe SM, Chertow GM, Parfrey PS, Kubo Y, Block GA, Correa-Rotter R, et al. Cinacalcet, fibroblast growth factor-23, and cardiovascular disease in hemodialysis: the evaluation of cinacalcet HCl therapy to lower cardiovascular events (EVOLVE) trial. Circulation. 2015;132:27–39.

Parfrey PS, Drüeke TB, Block GA, Correa-Rotter R, Floege J, Herzog CA, et al. The effects of cinacalcet in older and younger patients on hemodialysis: the evaluation of cinacalcet HCl therapy to lower cardiovascular events (EVOLVE) trial. Clin J Am Soc Nephrol. 2015;10:791–9.

Disorders of the Serum Sodium Concentration

15

Julian L. Seifter and Hsin-Yun Chang

Contents

J. L. Seifter (✉)
Brigham and Women's Hospital, Department of Medicine,
Boston, MA, USA
e-mail: jseifter@bwh.harvard.edu

H.-Y. Chang
National Cheng Kung University Hospital, Department of Family
Medicine, Tainan City, Taiwan

© Springer Nature Switzerland AG 2020
R. K. Garg et al. (eds.), *Handbook of Inpatient Endocrinology*,
https://doi.org/10.1007/978-3-030-38976-5_15

Abbreviations

ACE	Angiotensin-converting enzyme
ADH	Antidiuretic hormone
ANP	Atrial natriuretic peptide
AQP2	Aquaporin type 2
AVP	Arginine vasopressin
CHF	Congestive heart failure
CRH	Corticotropin-releasing hormone
ECF	Extracellular fluid
FES	Flame emission spectrophotometer
ICF	Intracellular fluid
ODS	Osmotic demyelination syndrome
RAAS	Renin-angiotensin-aldosterone system
SIADH	Syndrome of inappropriate antidiuresis hormone (SIADH)
SNS	Sympathetic nervous system

Basic Physiology of Sodium and Water Balance

The concentrations of Na^+, the most abundant extracellular fluid (ECF) cation, and K^+, the major intracellular cation, determine the osmolality of total body water. More than 90% of the total osmotic content of the ECF is accounted for by Na^+ and its accompanying anions, principally Cl^- and HCO_3^-.

Plasma osmolality can be seen as that of total body water since osmolality of almost all body compartments is the same; we then have the equation shown below:

$$\text{Plasma osmolality} = \frac{Extracellular + Intracellular\ solutes}{Total\ body\ water}$$
$$= \frac{2\left[Na^+ + K^+\right]}{Total\ body\ water} \simeq 2 \times \left[Na^+\right]$$

Therefore, plasma $[Na^+] \simeq (Na^+ + K^+)$/total body water.

Na^+ content is determined by dietary intake and regulated excretion independent of water regulatory mechanisms in order to maintain an adequate blood pressure and plasma volume required for perfusion of tissues. The state of total body potassium is also a reflection of diet and regulated excretion that determines cellular volume. Since most cell membranes are highly permeable to water, the regulation of osmolality usually depends on water balance.

Plasma $[Na^+]$ is kept within a narrow range of 135–145 mmol/kg (~mEq/L); an even narrower range of ~2% difference in an individual is often observed. Despite constantly changing dietary intake of salt and water, this finely regulated homeostatic control is due to an important thirst mechanism and renal regulation by means of the rapid stimulated release of the posterior pituitary peptide hormone, arginine vasopressin (AVP) , when conserving water is required and the rapid degradation of AVP in states of water excess. In turn, adequate ability to concentrate urine to maximal levels in humans (~1200 mOsm/kg) requires intact tubular functions of the kidney, adequate salt and protein diets to allow for urinary concentrating ability, and a complex system of countercurrent exchange and multiplication.

The systems of regulating osmolality and extracellular volume (and therefore blood pressure) are mostly different, but they intersect in the setting of changes in volume expansion or depletion (Fig. 15.1).

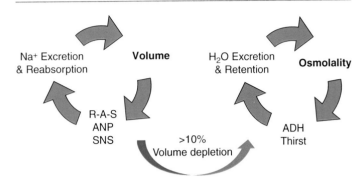

Fig. 15.1 The systems regulating osmolality and volume are mostly different but interact in the setting of changes in volume. ADH secretion is stimulated as systemic osmolality is raised above a threshold level of 285 mOsm/kg. Over the physiologic range of effective circulating volume, ADH levels are determined almost entirely by plasma osmolality. However, extracellular volume depletion of 10% or greater also significantly influences ADH levels. Both increase in plasma osmolality and decrease in extracellular volume stimulate the "thirst center." The sympathetic nerve system (SNS) and renin-angiotensin system (RAS) , on the other hand, respond to smaller decrements of extracellular volume changes. In excessive fluid loss, baroreceptors stimulate sympathetic activity to the kidneys, triggering vasoconstriction mainly in efferent arterioles to maintain GFR as well as renin secretion and Na^+ reabsorption along nephron. In renin-angiotensin system (RAS), angiotensin II also causes vasoconstriction in efferent arteriole to maintain GFR and promotes aldosterone secretion so as to stimulate increased Na^+ reabsorption. Atrial natriuretic peptide (ANP) can be seen as the counter regulatory system for the RAS, causing systemic vasodilation and increased Na^+ and water excretion in response to extracellular volume expansion

Osmoregulation of ADH

The absence or presence of ADH is the major physiologic determinant of urinary water excretion or retention. ADH secretion is stimulated as systemic osmolality is raised above a threshold level of 285 mOsm/kg. Decreases in blood pressure and intravascular fluid volume also stimulate ADH release and thirst but in a less sensitive manner. In addition, there are other non-osmotic stimuli that activate ADH release, including hypoxemia, nausea, stress (pain, emotion, exercise), alcohol, serotonin, and multiple drugs.

ADH acts on renal V_2 receptors to increase permeability to water in the collecting ducts, permeability to urea in the inner medullary collecting ducts, and reabsorption of NaCl by the thick ascending limb, distal tubule, and collecting duct.

Increases in plasma osmolality or decrease in volume stimulates the "thirst centers," which is located in the same regions of hypothalamus as involved with ADH secretion. Other thirst receptors are located in the oropharynx. Osmotic threshold for triggering thirst is higher than that for ADH secretion (295 vs. 285 mOsm/kg). ADH will be suppressed by hypotonicity once ADH threshold is reached. The secretion of ADH reduces water loss in urine in the setting of water deprivation, and the ADH threshold being lower than that of thirst prevents an otherwise continuous cycle of polyuria and polydipsia. In diabetes insipidus, ADH is either inadequate in concentration or absent. The major sign is potentially massive dilute urine production, which becomes serious if water consumption is not available. On the other hand, in the syndrome of inappropriate antidiuretic hormone secretion (SIADH) , ingestion of water does not adequately suppress ADH, and the urine remains more concentrated than expected.

Relation Between Plasma Osmolality and Sodium Concentration

Osmolality is a measure of the number of particles present in solution and is independent of the size or weight of the particles. Plasma osmolality (P_{osm}) can be estimated as the calculated osmolarity (P_{osm}):

$$P_{osm} = 2 \times \left[Na^+ \right] + glucose\left(mg/dL\right)/18 \\ + blood\ urea\ nitrogen\left(mg/dL\right)/2.8$$

The multiple of 2 for the plasma sodium concentration accounts for the osmotic contribution of its accompanying anions in the extracellular fluid. The concentrations of glucose and blood urea nitrogen (BUN) being divided by 18 and 2.8 are to convert the frequently measured units of mg/dL into mmol/L.

In healthy subjects, glucose and urea are both present in low concentrations and are ineffective osmoles because they can cross cell membranes. Therefore, sodium acts as the main effective osmole in plasma, and the equation can be simplified as $P_{osm} \simeq 2 \times [Na^+]$.

Hyponatremia can result from either loss of Na^+ and K^+ or increase in total body water due to retention of ingested or infused water. Solute losses from vomiting or diarrhea typically occur in fluids that are iso-osmotic to plasma, which do not lead to changes in plasma $[Na^+]$. Only if the fluids are replaced with ingested water will hyponatremia occur because ECF depletion leads to non-osmotic ADH release. Therefore, the cause for nearly all cases of hyponatremia is abnormal water retention leading to excess water in relation to solute. On the other hand, continuous water loss, and sometimes sodium overload, accounts for the occurrence of hypernatremia.

Relation Between Osmolality and Tonicity

Plasma tonicity, also called the effective plasma osmolality, equals the sum of the concentrations of the solutes which have the capacity to exert an osmotic force across the membrane. It reflects the concentration of solutes that do not easily cross cell membranes and therefore determines the transcellular distribution of water between the cells and the ECF.

Fluid expansion and depletion contributing to disorders of serum $[Na^+]$ are summarized in Table 15.1. Hyponatremia occurs when a defect in urinary dilution is combined with water intake that exceeds the ability to quantitatively excrete enough water, while hypernatremia develops when there is loss of water in excess of sodium without appropriate water intake or by expansion with hypertonic fluids. Note that both hyponatremia and hypernatremia can be associated with increased, decreased, or normal ECF volume. This is because ECF depletion, which always accompanies Na^+ loss, may be due to losses of Na^+ as hypertonic fluid (hyponatremia), isotonic fluid (normonatremia), or hypotonic fluid (hypernatremia). The expansion syndromes similarly accompany gains

Table 15.1   Syndromes of fluid expansion and depletion

	Hematocrit	[Protein]	[Na⁺]	ECF volume	ICF volume	Examples
Expansion						
Na > H₂O	↓	↓	↑	↑	↓	Hypertonic expansion (hypertonic NaHCO₃ or NaCl infusion)
Na = H₂O	↓	↓	–	↑	–	Isotonic expansion (saline infusion)
Na < H₂O	↓	↓	↓	↑	↑	Hypotonic expansion (1/2 NS infusion)
Depletion						
Na > H₂O	↑	↑	↑	↓	↑	Hypertonic depletion (diabetes insipidus)
Na = H₂O	↑	↑	–	↓	–	Isotonic depletion (sweating, vomiting)
Na < H₂O	↑	↑	↓	↓	↓	Hypotonic depletion (salt-wasting)

of hypotonic fluids (hyponatremia), isotonic fluids (normonatremia), or hypertonic fluids (hypenatremia).

Initial Approach to Dysnatremia

Direct history and initial physical examination often provide useful information and guide the subsequent diagnostic approach. For example, a history of fluid loss from vomiting, diarrhea, and diuretic therapy, or signs of extracellular fluid volume depletion such as decreased skin turgor and orthostatic or persistent hypotension, may suggest hypovolemic state. Inadequate fluid intake or poor diet, presence or absence of thirst and polyuria, medical history consistent with malignancy, heart failure, recent surgery, and certain medication use including antiepileptics and antipsychotics may all direct toward determining the causes of dysnatremias and further management. Routine laboratory chemistries may provide certain information, e.g., renal dysfunction and hyperkalemia suggesting hypoaldosteronism. Further investigation should include urine chemistries. Imaging may be necessary to detect or confirm associated etiology. Note that dysnatremias are often multifactorial and clinical evaluation should consider all possible causes.

Clinical Features of Dysnatremia and Cell Adaptation

The symptoms of dysnatremia are mainly neurological due to the effects on the central nervous system. In hyponatremia, a fall in plasma tonicity results in osmotic water movement from the ECF into the cells, including brain cells, and leads to neurologic dysfunction. In hypernatremia, there is an osmotic water movement out of the brain cells due to increased plasma tonicity. Symptoms of dysnatremia are associated with the rapidity of the changes in the plasma sodium concentration. Nausea and malaise are common in early stage, while severe symptoms including seizures, brainstem herniation, and coma may develop when dysnatremia is acute or if a chronic condition is corrected too rapidly.

When encountering changes in plasma tonicity, the brain attempts to adapt to hyponatremia by losing intracellular solutes (potassium and organics, e.g., amines, polyols, amino acids, glycerophosphocholine) and to hypernatremia by increasing intracellular solutes. The process of cell adaptation may be completed in 1–2 days with major implications for therapy. Brain cell volume may normalize within 1–2 days despite the continued change in osmolality and may change abruptly if osmolality is corrected instantly.

This can explain why patients with chronic dysnatremia are less likely to develop severe neurological deficits upon presentation but are predisposed to cerebral edema and seizures if encountering overcorrection of plasma sodium concentration (> 8–10 m*M*/d).

Diagnostic Approach to Hyponatremia

Is the Hyponatremia "True or Fictitious"?

Hyponatremia is defined as a serum sodium level of less than 135 mmol/L. Decreased serum sodium often reflects a hypotonic state; however, hyponatremia may also occur with iso-osmotic or hyperosmotic plasma. It is prerequisite to confirm hypotonic and exclude non-hypotonic hyponatremia (Fig. 15.2).

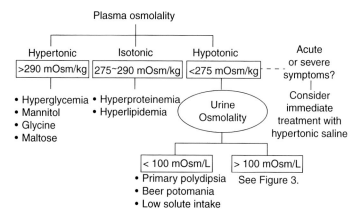

Fig. 15.2 Establish the type of hyponatremia by first measuring plasma osmolality, and obtain urine osmolality to assess ADH activity in the hypotonic hyponatremic patients. Note that a rapid decline in plasma sodium over 24–48 h is a medical emergency and requires acute intervention

- Iso-osmotic hyponatremia is caused factitiously by hyperproteinemia and hyperlipidemia, as solids that may contribute to more than the normal volume of plasma (>10%) and if the measurement is made by indirect potentiometry, a method of diluting of serum.

The laboratory artifact is known as *pseudohyponatremia*. Excluding factitious hyponatremia requires a measure of serum osmolality or the Na⁺ concentration by direct potentiometry (undiluted sample) usually on a blood gas analyzer.

Is the Hyponatremia Associated with Hypo-osmolairty

The presence of solutes which do not penetrate cell membranes such as glucose (in the absence of insulin) and mannitol decreases plasma sodium by shifting water from intracellular to extracellular space. A decrease in serum [Na⁺] of 2.4 mmol/L occurs for every 100 mg/dL increase in plasma glucose particularly when glucose is greater than 400 mg/dL. Estimates of the serum sodium concentration corrected for the presence of hyperglycemia can be obtained from the equations:

$$\text{Corrected serum}\left[Na^{+} \right] = \text{measured}\left[Na^{+} \right] + 2.4$$
$$\times \frac{glucose\left(\dfrac{mg}{dL} \right) - 100\left(\dfrac{mg}{dL} \right)}{100\left(\dfrac{mg}{dL} \right)}$$

Plasma osmolality can alsobe increased by certain solutes including urea, ethanol, methanol, and ethylene glycol. These solutes are cell membrane permeable and do not translocate water into the intra- or extracellular space. Their presence does not cause hyponatremia but can lead to a normal or high measured plasma osmolality in a hyponatremic patient from other cause. These patients should be approached as having a hypotonic disorder given their decreased effective plasma tonicity.

Is the ADH Activity Appropriately Suppressed?

• Obtain urine osmolality to assess ADH activity in the hypotonic hyponatremic patient.

To evaluate hyponatremia, urine osmolality is used to assess
ADH activity. The development of hyponatremia along with
hypo-osmolality is often caused by underlying disorders affecting
the renal diluting mechanism. Such patients have a greater than
maximally dilute urine, which is 50–100 mOsm/kg, unless hypo-
osmolality fails to fully suppress ADH release (the reset osmostat). When the urine osmolality is < 100 mOsm/kg, indicating
maximally dilute urine, the hyponatremia is primarily caused by
excess water intake or low solute intake. Psychogenic polydipsia
and beer potomania are classic examples. This example demonstrates the difference between urinary dilution, a measure of concentration, and excretion of quantitatively enough dilute urine,
measured by free water clearance rate, in ml/min.

Diagnostic Categories of Hyponatermia Based on the Extracellular Volume

Ingestion of a normal diet in a healthy subject results in the excretion of approximately 600 mOsm of solute per day, which includes
primarily sodium, potassium salts, and urea. If the minimum urine
osmolality is 50 mOsmol/kg, the maximum urine output will be
12 L/day. In beer drinkers (beer potomania) or those on a very
poor diet, there is little solute (low sodium, potassium, or protein)
in the diet. Also the carbohydrate load in beer may further suppress endogenous protein breakdown. Therefore, daily solute
excretion may be less than 150 mOsm, and hyponatremia occurs
if daily fluid intake exceeds 3 L/day. Patients with hyponatremia
due to beer potomania and low solute intake respond rapidly to
intravenous saline and a resumption of a normal diet. However,
patients with beer potomania are at high risk of developing
osmotic demyelinating syndrome (ODS) due to the associated
hypokalemia, alcoholism, malnutrition, and potentially overcor-
rected plasma sodium concentration.

Primary polydipsia occurs when more hypotonic fluid is consumed than excreted in a maximally dilute urine. It is characterized by increase in thirst and is most often seen in patients with psychiatric illnesses. Changes in plasma osmolality play the most important role in regulating ADH secretion. Osmolality is sensed by osmoreceptors in the anterior hypothalamus, which shrink or swell in response to changes in osmolality. Decrease in plasma osmolality will cause osmoreceptors to swell and thereby decrease ADH secretion. In primary polydipsia, the patients continue to drink until the thirst threshold, causing fall in plasma osmolality suppressing ADH secretion with diuresis and subsequently continued stimulation of thirst. An acute water load of 3–4 L may cause fatal hyponatremia even though the urine is maximally dilute.

- Determine the patient's volume status and obtain urine sodium concentration.

In the patient with hypotonic hyponatremia whose urine is not dilute (>100 mOsm/L), an assessment of the ECF volume has been proposed to help further differentiate the underlying causes (Fig. 15.3). However, in clinical practice, a mixed process may occur, or a hypovolemic state often presents as clinical euvolemia, making such classification debatable. Measuring urine Na^+ and K^+ concentrations is therefore always essential. Calculations of electrolyte-free water clearance are recommended ($C_{H2O} = V - (U_{Na} + U_K)V/P_{Na}$). Note that since water is coming from TBW, both Na and K are required. This equation enables independent calculations of isotonic and free water excretion. It is helpful in diagnosis and treatment. For example, a positive C_{H2O} and hypernatremia suggests diabetes insipidus. C_{H2O} also improves management as it informs about ongoing urinary losses. While deficits are calculated based on an abnormal serum $[Na^+]$ and must be corrected at a safe rate, ongoing losses will lead to a deficit if not replaced quantitatively. Another advantage of calculating C_{H2O} is in the choice of management strategy. Thus, if the urine was hypertonic in a hyponatremic patient, giving saline may make a patient with SIADH more hyponatremic. Also, in the same patient, a large negative value for C_{H2O} predicts that fluid restric-

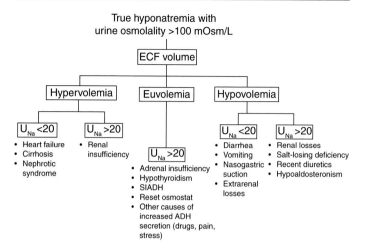

Fig. 15.3 Determine the patient's volume status and obtain urine sodium concentration for further diagnosis

tion may be inadequate. In that case, treatment with a loop diuretic may be helpful to diminish the maximal urine osmolality, or cautious use of hypertonic saline may be required. When using a loop diuretic in a patient with hypertonic urine, it is necessary to recalculate C_{H2O} to assure success in creating hypotonic urine.

Hypervolemic Hyponatremia

When hyponatremia occurs with excess ECF volume, both total body sodium and total body water are increased, with total body water being increased to a greater extent. In this setting, the edematous state may be due to congestive heart failure (CHF), cirrhosis, nephrotic syndrome, or advanced kidney disease.

In CHF, cirrhosis, and nephrotic syndrome, a decreased effective circulating arterial volume leads to increased ADH secretion. Aquaporin 2 (AQP2) water channels may also be increased, resulting in decreased water clearance. Urinary sodium level is often very low (may be < 10 mmol/L) in these cases, as renin-angiotensin-aldosterone system (RAAS) increases sodium retention. However, sodium retention can be obscured by diuretics, which are often used concomitantly to treat such patients.

In advanced renal insufficiency, hyponatremia is associated with water intakes exceeding the ability to excrete equivalent volumes, and the minimum urine osmolality can rise to as high as 200–250 mOsmol/L. A decrement in GFR and the impairment of free water excretion with increase in thirst contribute to the retention of ingested water and the development of a hypervolemic hyponatremic state. Hypervolemic hyponatremia due to CHF will often respond to improved therapy of the underlying cardiomyopathy, e.g., following the institution or intensification of angiotensin-converting enzyme (ACE) inhibition.

Hypovolemic Hyponatremia

As noted earlier, plasma sodium concentration can be determined by:

$$2\left(Na^+ + K^+\right)/\,Total\;body\;water$$

The loss of sodium and possibly potassium may contribute to hyponatremia, if these losses are not accompanied by parallel decrements in total body water. When there are substantial fluid losses, from either renal or extrarenal sources, volume contraction stimulates secretion of ADH. If these losses are replenished with water or hypotonic fluids, hyponatremia will result. We know that over the physiologic range of effective circulating volume, ADH levels are determined almost entirely by plasma osmolality. However, volume depletion of 10% or greater will significantly influence ADH levels. Therefore, in the presence of hypovolemia, ADH is secreted with subsequent water retention even in the presence of hypotonicity. On examination, a low jugular venous pressure, decreased skin turgor, orthostatic hypotension, and tachycardia may be noticed. A urinary sodium concentration of less than 20 mEq/L indicates a normal renal response to volume depletion by conserving sodium, and an extrarenal loss is suggested. Vomiting or diarrhea, or fluid losses into third spaces such as burns or pancreatitis, can all lead to hypovolemia. The urinary sodium concentration can be as low as <10 mEq/L. However, in patients with vomiting and metabolic alkalosis presenting bicarbonaturia, urinary sodium concentration can be greater than 20 mEq/L, while urinary chloride concentration will be low since bicarbonate anion dominates. Both the sodium and chloride concentrations can be as high as 40 meq/L in hypovolemic hyponatremic patients with renal salt losses, which is most commonly seen with diuretic therapy if the urine electrolytes are measured while the effect of the diuretic is still present. The variation in the hyponatremia risk relates to the site of action in different diuretics. Loop diuretics interfere with sodium chloride (NaCl) reabsorption in the thick ascending limb of the loop of Henle by impairing the accumulation of NaCl in the medulla. Although the loop diuretic can increase ADH levels by inducing volume depletion, responsiveness to ADH is diminished because of the impairment in the medullary gradient. As a result, water retention and the development of hyponatremia will be limited. The thiazides, in comparison, act in the cortex of distal tubule and do not interfere with medullary function or with ADH-induced urinary concentration in volume depletion. In addition to water retention, increased sodium and potassium excretion due to the diuretic as well as enhanced water retention can result in the excretion of electrolyte-rich urine with a sodium plus potassium concentration higher than that of the plasma and directly promote the development of hyponatremia regardless of water intake. Hyponatremia related to use of thiazides begins soon after initiation and is often evident within 14 days. Furosemide-related hyponatremia tends to occur after many months of therapy, often when an intercurrent illness develops in polydipsic patients.

If urinary sodium concentration higher than 20 mEq/L accompanies hyperkalemia and elevated plasma urea and creatinine, hypoaldosteronism should be suspected.

Hypovolemic hyponatremia responds to volume restoration with isotonic normal saline – most importantly, the recognition of underlying etiology needs to be identified. It should be obvious that the urinary chemistries in hypovolemic hyponatremia and hypervolemic hyponatremia, as in CHF, are similar. The one hor-

monal difference in the plasma may be a high BNP (B-type natriuretic peptide) in CHF, whereas it will be low in hypovolemia.

Euvolemic Hyponatremia

Euvolemic hyponatremia is the most heterogeneous and commonly encountered hyponatremia in hospitalized patients. Patients
may have slightly excessive volume in the absence of edema, and
it may be hard to distinguish from hypovolemia. Urine chemistry
again is vital to differentiation, and sodium is expected to be
>20 mEq/L. Euvolemic hyponatremia can occur in any of the set-
tings mentioned above and is seen in other scenarios. The question often arises as to why patients with water overload but not
salt and water overload do not get edema. One reason is that only
6% of a water load expands the plasma volume as most water goes
into cells. By the time water was expanded enough to cause
edema, life-threatening hyponatremia would develop. A second
reason is that an acute water load expands the plasma volume
enough to cause a mild, acute natriuresis. But distinctively the
cause of edema in ECF expansion is raised intravascular volume
and pressure due to the gravitational effect on the veins. The result
is an increased intracapillary hydrostatic pressure gradient in
dependent areas such as lower extremities. In contrast, hypo-
osmotic expansion with water will affect oncotic forces throughout the body, and there will be no effect of gravity to increase
Starling forces in dependent areas.

Secondary adrenal insufficiency due to pituitary disease may
lead to euvolemic hyponatremia, while decreased aldosterone in
primary adrenal insufficiency causes hypovolemic hyponatremia.
In either primary or secondary adrenal insufficiency, glucocorticoid deficiency leads to co-secretion of corticotropin-releasing
hormone (CRH) and ADH by the paraventricular nuclei in the
hypothalamus. Impaired water excretion with reduced water
delivery to the collecting ducts is also associated with
glucocorticoid deficiency. Hydrocortisone replacement in these
patients will reduce ADH secretion and therefore normalize its
response to osmolality.

In patients with hypothyroidism, the cardiac output is often reduced and may be the non-osmotic stimuli to ADH release, while the concomitant reduction in GFR leads to diminished free water excretion. Hyponatremia in this case can be reversed by treatment with levothyroxine.

The syndrome of inappropriate antidiuretic hormone (SIADH) is a common cause of euvolemic hyponatremia in hospitalized patients. The diagnosis is made mainly by excluding other causes and can be summarized in Table 15.2. In normal individuals, plasma ADH levels are very low when the plasma osmolality is below 280 mOsmo/kg, permitting the excretion of ingested water. ADH levels increase progressively as the plasma osmolality rises above 280 mOsm/kg, and the higher the plasma ADH, the more concentrated the urine. In most patients with SIADH, ingestion of water does not adequately suppress ADH, and the urine remains concentrated. Sustained increases in ADH limit distal renal tubular transport, thereby preserving a relatively hypervolemic state with hyponatremia. Such patients are not euvolemic but rather subclinically volume-expanded. Serum uric acid is often low (<4 mg/dL) in patients with SIADH, while hyperuricemia is often seen in patients with hypovolemic hyponatremia. Common causes of SIADH include pulmonary disease, central nervous system disorders, and malignancies, most commonly in small-cell lung carcinoma. Patients with euvolemic hyponatremia due to SIADH may respond to successful treatment of the underlying cause. However, not all causes of SIADH are immediately reversible, and pharmacologic therapy may be necessary at certain point. Oral tolvaptan, the ADH V_2 antagonist, may be considered

Table 15.2 Diagnostic criteria for SIADH

Decreased serum osmolality (<275 mOsm/kg)
Increased urine osmolality (>100 mOsm/kg)
Clinical euvolemia
Increased urinary sodium concentration (>40 mmol/L) under normal salt and water intake
Absence of adrenal, thyroid, pituitary, or renal insufficiency or recent diuretic use

in significant and uncontrolled SIADH which is not responsive to the treatment with water restriction, oral furosemide, and salt tablets.

The "reset osmostat" is sometimes considered a variant of SIADH, in which the threshold for ADH secretion is reset downward so that ADH is secreted at a lower value instead of beyond 280–285 mOsm/kg as in most individuals. Diagnosing reset osmostat is a diagnosis of exclusion. Individuals with reset osmostat should be able to concentrate and dilute the urine appropriately, and a water challenge should result in a dilute urine (<100 mOsm/kg), while a water deprivation test results in a concentrated urine. Reset osmostat often occurs in pregnancy, malnutrition, and neurologic conditions such as epilepsy and paraplegia. A patient initially diagnosed with SIADH will sometimes be proven with virtually reset osmostat when it becomes apparent that fluid restriction does not successfully raise the serum sodium level.

Management of Hyponatremia

The major considerations in managing hyponatremia are:

1. The presence or absence, as well as severity, of symptoms
2. The duration of the disorder
3. Recognizing the underlying cause

Patients with acute hyponatremia (with hyponatremia developing within 48 h) may present with symptoms ranging from headache, nausea, or vomiting to lethargy, seizures, or even coma and are also at greater risk of developing permanent neurologic sequelae. Patients with chronic hyponatremia (present for >48 h) are less likely to have severe symptoms. The risk of seizures remains low until the serum sodium concentration falls below 115 meq/L, and rarely patients may even be awake and talking with a serum sodium of <100 meq/L. However, patients with chronic hyponatremia are at greater risk for osmotic demyelinating syndrome (ODS) if plasma sodium concentration is corrected by >8–10 mM within the first 24 h or by >18 mM within the first 48 h. In contrast, in acute hyponatremia, overly rapid correction is less of a concern since the brain has not yet adapted completely to the hypotonic environment. Clinically, it may be unclear which treatments should be applied or what increases in plasma sodium concentration we should pursue. While treatment can be diagnosis specific, a single infusion of 150 mL 3% hypertonic saline may be suggested to avoid further drop in plasma sodium concentration. Nevertheless, frequent monitoring of plasma sodium concentration during corrective therapy is always crucial because a variation in the volume and electrolyte content of the urine produced concomitantly may also have an impact.

Aggressive therapy to rapidly raise the serum sodium with hypertonic saline is indicated when patients present with severe symptoms such as seizures or obtundation or acute hyponatremia even with mild symptoms. The goal of such therapy is to rapidly increase the serum sodium by 4–6 mEq/L over a period of several hours. Note that the increase in serum sodium should not exceed 8 mEq/L in any given 24-h period.

Patients who are asymptomatic or have mild to moderate symptoms with even acute or severe hyponatremia (i.e., serum sodium $\leq$ 120 mEq/L) do not require emergent therapy, and the goal is to slowly raise the serum sodium and alleviate symptoms. In general, raising the serum sodium by 4–6 mEq/L should improve a patient's symptoms. Calculating a proper dose of 3% saline can be reasoned as follows: 3% saline has 513 meq/L NaCl (~0.5 meq/ml). Total body water is ~50% body weight in kilogram. Therefore, giving 1 ml/kg body weight will raise the [Na$^+$] by 1 meq/L. Thus, to raise the serum [Na$^+$] by 1 meq/L over 4 h in a 70 kg man, one would give 3% saline at a rate of 70 ml/hr for 4 h.

Once the corrective therapy has been established and initiated, treatment should be directed at the underlying disease. In the case of overcorrection of hyponatremia (raising the Na$^+$ greater than 8 mEq/L/day), water can be given as D5W with an amount to lower the Na$^+$ to a value appropriate for the time elapsed. In cases where large elecrolyte free water clearance may correct hyponatremia too rapidly (as after saline given to a patient with

hypovolemic hyponatremia) SC or IV DDAVP may be administered to clamp the urine output to low levels. Then the administration of 3% saline allows correction at an appropriate rate.
Since 3% saline is ~0.5 meq Na+/ml and total body water is ~0.5
times the body weight, it follows that administering 3% saline at
1 ml/kg body weight will raise the serum Na+ by 1 meq/L.

Diagnostic Approach to Hypernatremia

Hypernatremia is defined as an increase in the plasma Na^+ concentration to >145 mmol/L, reflecting losses of water via both
renal and nonrenal routes in excess of sodium and potassium. Net
water loss accounts for the majority. In order for hypernatremia to
occur, either ADH function or thirst mechanism must be impaired,
and limited access to water is often involved. In those who are
alert and have an intact thirst mechanism and adequate access to
water, persistent hypernatremia should rarely occur. The higher
the GFR, or proximal tubule sodium, glucose, or urea delivery, the
higher the urine volume.

A detailed history and physical examination often reveal the
underlying causes of hypernatremia. In the elderly, it is often due
to water losses without adequate replacement due to altered mental status or limited access. Still, further investigation may be necessary when etiology is unclear (Table 15.3).

As in hyponatremia, hypernatremia must be considered along
with ECF status.

Hypervolemic Hypernatremia

If hypervolemia is present, sodium gains from hypertonic fluid
administration or mineralocorticoid excess must be considered.
Urine sodium concentration, if obtained, is often >20 mmol/L. The
urine may in fact be hypertonic, though rarely maximally concentrated due to washout of the medullary solute gradient. However,
the net hypertonic salt intake must exceed the net hypertonic salt
output. It is often asked whether someone can survive by drinking

Table 15.3 Common causes of hypernatremia

Dehydration (nonrenal loss)
Insensible losses
Gastrointestinal losses
Primary hypodipsia
Sodium gains
Hypertonic sodium load
Hyperaldosteronism
Cushing's syndrome
Osmotic diuresis
Glucosuria
High urea in high-protein tube feedings
Mannitol
Water diuresis
Central diabetes insipidus
Nephrogenic diabetes insipidus

ocean water. Sea water is about 1000 meq Na^+ and Cl^-. The bowel can only absorb isosmotically. Thus, drinking seawater will increase isotonic salt water reabsorption, but the remaining hypertonic salt will induce severe isotonic diarrhea. The total body water will decrease. But the serum Na^+ will rise, dehydrating cells while expanding the ECF. The result is hypertonic expansion. Urine osm and tonicity will rise (high ADH) and polyuria will result.

Hypovolemic/Euvolemic Hypernatremia

There may be evident history of extrarenal losses, e.g., increased. insensible loss, gastrointestinal loss, or burn. Minimum volume of maximally concentrated urine with urine osmolality >700 mOsm/kg and urinary sodium concentration <10 mmol/L may further support the diagnosis. If the urine osmolality appears less than 300 mOsm/kg, the patient is suspected with either central or nephrogenic diabetes insipidus, which can be distinguished by the administration of exogenous ADH (dDAVP), followed by monitoring of the urine osmolality and volume every 30 min over the next 2 h.

If the urine osmolality is intermediate (between 300 and 800 mOsmol/kg), the hypernatremia may be due to diabetes insipidus or an osmotic diuresis. Such patients can be differentiated by measuring the total solute excretion. As mentioned earlier, ingestion of a normal diet in a healthy subject results in the excretion of approximately 600 mOsm (600–900 mOsm) of solute per day. A value above 900 mOsm/day suggests a significant contribution from increased solute excretion, indicating osmotic diuresis resulting from possibly glucosuria, mannitol, or high solute loads. If an osmotic diuresis is not present, a workup to rule out diabetes insipidus should be performed.

Management of Hypernatremia

The water deficit in the hypernatremic patient can be estimated from the following formula:

$$\text{Free water deficit} = \text{Current total body water} \times \left(\frac{Serum\left[Na^+ \right]}{140} - 1 \right)$$

Total body water is estimated by multiplying weight in kilograms by 0.6 for men and by 0.5 for women. The formulas estimate the amount of water required to have been lost to raise the serum sodium from a relatively normal level of 140 to the hypernatremic value. To correct the [Na$^+$] would require replacing that amount of water. Chronic hypernatremia (>48 h) or hypernatremia of unknown duration should be corrected at a safe rate at which the serum sodium concentration should be lowered no more than 10 meq/L per day to avoid cerebral edema caused by excess fall in serum [Na$^+$]. As for acute hypernatremia, serum sodium level should be corrected over the next 24 h. Concurrent electrolyte disturbances should not be ignored and must be replenished accordingly.

Meanwhile, ongoing free water losses, including losses in sweat, stool, dilute urinary, or gastrointestinal tract, must be replaced as well. In addition, this formula does not include combined sodium and water loss, as in diarrhea or an osmotic diuresis.

Suggested Reading

Adrogue HJ, Madias NE. Hypernatremia. N Engl J Med. 2000;342(20):1493–9.

Ashraf N, Locksley R, Arieff AI. Thiazide-induced hyponatremia associated with death or neurologic damage in outpatients. Am J Med. 1981;70(6):1163–8.

Ayus JC, Caputo D, Bazerque F, Heguilen R, Gonzalez CD, Moritz ML. Treatment of hyponatremic encephalopathy with a 3% sodium chloride protocol: a case series. Am J Kidney Dis. 2015;65(3):435–42.

Chung HM, Kluge R, Schrier RW, Anderson RJ. Clinical assessment of extracellular fluid volume in hyponatremia. Am J Med. 1987;83(5):905–8.

Hillier TA, Abbott RD, Barrett EJ. Hyponatremia: evaluating the correction factor for hyperglycemia. Am J Med. 1999;106(4):399–403.

Hoorn EJ, Zietse R. Hyponatremia revisited: translating physiology to practice. Nephron Physiol. 2008;108(3):p46–59.

List AF, Hainsworth JD, Davis BW, Hande KR, Greco FA, Johnson DH. The syndrome of inappropriate secretion of antidiuretic hormone (SIADH) in small-cell lung cancer. J Clin Oncol. 1986;4(8):1191–8.

Sahay M, Sahay R. Hyponatremia: a practical approach. Indian J Endocrinol Metab. 2014;18(6):760–71.

Sanghvi SR, Kellerman PS, Nanovic L. Beer potomania: an unusual cause of hyponatremia at high risk of complications from rapid correction. Am J Kidney Dis. 2007;50(4):673–80.

Sterns RH. Formulas for fixing serum sodium: curb your enthusiasm. Clin Kidney J. 2016;9(4):527–9.

Sterns RH, Cappuccio JD, Silver SM, Cohen EP. Neurologic sequelae after treatment of severe hyponatremia: a multicenter perspective. J Am Soc Nephrol. 1994;4(8):1522–30.

Sterns RH, Hix JK, Silver S. Treatment of hyponatremia. Curr Opin Nephrol Hypertens. 2010;19(5):493–8.

Szatalowicz VL, Miller PD, Lacher JW, Gordon JA, Schrier RW. Comparative effect of diuretics on renal water excretion in hyponatraemic oedematous disorders. Clin Sci (Lond, England: 1979). 1982;62(2):235–8.

Verbalis JG, Adler S, Schrier RW, Berl T, Zhao Q, Czerwiec FS. Efficacy and safety of oral tolvaptan therapy in patients with the syndrome of inappropriate antidiuretic hormone secretion. Eur J Endocrinol. 2011;164(5):725–32.

Weisberg LS. Pseudohyponatremia: a reappraisal. Am J Med. 1989;86(3):315–8.

Inpatient Management of Hyperkalemia

16

Erika R. Drury and Bradley M. Denker

Contents

E. R. Drury
Division of Nephrology, Department of Medicine, University of
Rochester School of Medicine, Rochester, NY, USA
e-mail: erika_drury@urmc.rochester.edu

B. M. Denker (✉)
Beth Israel Deaconess Medical Center, Department of Medicine,
Nephrology Division and Harvard Medical School, Boston, MA, USA
e-mail: bdenker@bidmc.harvard.edu

© Springer Nature Switzerland AG 2020   189
R. K. Garg et al. (eds.), *Handbook of Inpatient Endocrinology*,
https://doi.org/10.1007/978-3-030-38976-5_16

Obtain Whole Blood Potassium in the Setting of Hemolysis, Thrombocytosis, or Marked Leukocytosis

Pseudohyperkalemia refers to an elevation in potassium that occurs after the blood specimen has been drawn and does not represent true hyperkalemia. This should be suspected when there are no electrocardiographic changes such as peaked T waves associated with elevated potassium levels (>6 mEq/L), when the laboratory measurements of potassium levels are widely varying, or when there is no apparent cause for the hyperkalemia. The most common cause of pseudohyperkalemia is hemolysis from the trauma of venipuncture, which leads to the release of potassium from hemolyzed cells. If the blood specimen has been hemolyzed, repeat the measurement. Patients with thrombocytosis (platelet count >500,000/mm^3) may exhibit pseudohyperkalemia. A small amount of potassium moves out of cells when blood clots, but more potassium may be released in the presence of thrombocytosis. Ask for a measurement of the *plasma* (whole blood) potassium (from a heparinized blood sample) which will reveal the true in vivo potassium levels in these patients. Patients with marked leukocytosis (white cell count >100/mm^3) may also exhibit hyperkalemia. Leukemic lymphocytes are fragile and may release potassium when exposed to heparin or shaken. To exclude these scenarios, whole blood potassium from a sample in a blood gas tube should be taken, or samples should be walked to the lab, respectively. If pseudohyperkalemia can be excluded, then further workup and management is indicated.

Evaluate Symptoms and EKG to Exclude Life-Threatening Hyperkalemia

The most dangerous effects of hyperkalemia are cardiac arrhythmias and ascending muscle weakness and paralysis. These usually occur when the plasma potassium concentration is >7 mEq/L but can occur at lower concentrations if the hyperkalemia is acute or in the presence of hypocalcemia or acidemia. When plasma potassium levels are >6 mEq/L, order an electrocardiogram and place the patient on continuous telemetry monitoring. ECG changes associated with hyperkalemia begin with peaking of the *T* waves and shortening of the QT interval followed by widening of the QRS complex and the *P* wave and finally the appearance of the sine wave pattern followed by ventricular fibrillation or asystole. Rapid increases in serum potassium cause more pronounced cardiac toxicity (e.g., in acute renal failure). Ascending muscle weakness and flaccid paralysis usually occur only when the plasma potassium concentration is > 8 mEq/L but can occur at lower levels in patients with the genetic disorder hyperkalemic periodic paralysis.

Order Calcium Gluconate (1–2 g IV) to Treat Severe Hyperkalemia

Patients with a serum potassium concentration > 6.5 mEq/L and those with ECG changes or with muscle weakness require immediate treatment with measures aimed at reversing the effects of hyperkalemia followed by therapies to remove potassium from the body. Rapidly acting therapies include calcium, insulin, and *β*-agonists. Calcium does not lower serum potassium levels but lowers the myocyte membrane threshold potential and protects against the toxic effects of hyperkalemia. Give 1–2 g IV calcium gluconate (90–180 mg of elemental calcium) over 2–3 min. This acts within minutes but lasts only about 30–60 min, so repeated doses may be needed while potassium-lowering therapy is being administered.

Order Insulin 10 Units Plus Glucose 40–60 g as IV Bolus or Albuterol Nebulizer 10–20 mg to Shift Potassium Intracellularly

Insulin administration lowers the serum potassium concentration by driving it intracellularly. The usual regimen is 10 units of regular insulin given with 25 g of glucose (i.e., one "amp" of D50). This will lower the potassium concentration by 1–2 mEq/L within 60 min and lasts up to 4 h. If needed, insulin and dextrose can be repeated every 2–4 h. Nebulized beta agonists (i.e., albuterol) also lead to redistribution of potassium intracellularly. Up to 10–20 mg of nebulized albuterol is needed to lower the serum potassium level, which is in contrast to the 2.5 mg albuterol dose that is used for bronchospasm. If albuterol is used, give at least five standard dose nebulizers. This acts within 30 min and lasts 2–4 h. While these rapidly acting therapies are given, measures aimed at removal of potassium from the body should be instituted. In patients with severely impaired renal function such as advanced chronic kidney disease or acute renal failure, dialysis is often needed. In patients with normal or only mildly impaired renal function, other methods of removing potassium may be employed which include loop diuretics and gastrointestinal cation exchangers.

Assess History, Physical Exam, and Other Laboratory Data to Determine the Source of Potassium Load and Defect in Renal Excretion

Once life-threatening hyperkalemia has been excluded or is being managed, a thoughtful approach to determining the etiology of the hyperkalemia will help guide the best treatment. Take a thorough history and review the patient's laboratory values and medications. In most cases, the etiology of the hyperkalemia is multifactorial, but an impairment in renal excretion is required for the development of hyperkalemia.

First, assess for increased potassium release from cells. There are many factors that can contribute to hyperkalemia as a result of increased release from cells. In patients with metabolic acidosis, buffering of excess hydrogen ions leads to potassium shift out of the cell. Check an arterial or venous blood gas and measure the serum bicarbonate concentration. States of hyperglycemia and insulin deficiency lead to hyperkalemia, such as occurs in diabetic ketoacidosis (although often these patients are total body potassium depleted and will develop hypokalemia after treatment). Increased tissue catabolism as occurs with tumor lysis can lead to massive release of potassium into the extracellular space. Obtain laboratory tests that can suggest tumor lysis including uric acid, phosphorus, lactate dehydrogenase (LDH), and calcium. Evaluate for a history of fall or traumatic injury which leads to muscle cell necrosis and the development of rhabdomyolysis and elevated creatine phosphokinase (CPK) levels. Digitalis overdose can cause hyperkalemia as a result of inhibition of the Na-K-ATPase pump. For some of these conditions, measures aimed at correcting the abnormalities can help reduce the hyperkalemia. If a metabolic acidosis is present, treat the underlying cause (lactic acidosis, diabetic ketoacidosis), and sodium bicarbonate may be used if the serum pH is <7.1. If hyperglycemia is present, correct this with appropriate insulin therapy.

Second, assess for decreased urinary excretion of potassium. Reduced urinary excretion of potassium is the predominant driver for sustained hyperkalemia. Potassium excretion requires an adequate number of nephrons (GFR) and urine flow with distal sodium delivery to promote urinary potassium excretion. Finally, aldosterone is required for potassium excretion. Estimation of the potassium concentration in the tubular fluid of the collecting duct, which reflects tubular potassium secretion, may be possible by calculating the trans-tubular potassium gradient (TTKG) ([urine potassium (mEq/L) × serum osm (mOsm/kg)]/[serum potassium (mEq/L) × urine osm (mOsm/kg)]).

Values of <7 may suggest inappropriate renal response to hyper-kalemia and aldosterone deficiency. However, many argue that the TTKG is not valid because the underlying assumption that osmoles are not reabsorbed in the medullary collecting duct is incorrect. Therefore, calculation of the TTKG should be used with caution and in combination with the entirety of a patient's clinical picture. There are three major causes of reduced urinary potassium excretion: renal failure, effective arterial volume depletion, and hypoaldosteronism. To assess for acute or chronic renal failure, check for elevations in the serum urea nitrogen and creatinine. Hyperkalemia can occur in states of effective arterial volume depletion as potassium excretion requires delivery of water and sodium to the distal tubule, which is impaired in these states. Look for physical examination findings of true volume depletion such as orthostatic vital sign changes, hypotension, tachycardia, and diminished skin turgor. Patients with hypervolemia secondary to heart failure or cirrhosis often exhibit effective arterial volume depletion, so exam findings of pulmonary edema and peripheral edema are helpful. In both of these states, urine sodium levels will be <20 mEq/L, unless a loop diuretic has been recently used. Finally, hypoaldosteronism is the result of either reduced aldosterone production or aldosterone resistance. Reduced aldosterone secretion can be caused by drugs such as angiotensin-converting enzyme (ACE) inhibitors, angiotensin II receptor blockers (ARB), nonsteroidal anti-inflammatory drugs (NSAID(s)), calcineurin inhibitors, and heparin. Aldosterone antagonists such as spironolactone and eplerenone directly inhibit potassium excretion, while potassium-sparing diuretics such as amiloride and triamterene block the aldosterone-responsive epithelial sodium channel that is necessary for creating the lumen-negative potential necessary for potassium secretion. If these drugs are not present and a diagnosis of hypoaldosteronism is suspected, check morning plasma renin activity and aldosterone concentrations. Hyporeninemic hypoaldosteronism is characterized by low renin activity, whereas in primary adrenal insufficiency and in enzyme deficiencies, the plasma renin activity is elevated. Hyporeninemic hypoaldosteronism is also known as type IV renal tubular acidosis and can be seen in patients with diabetes and tubular disorders.

Order Intravenous Loop Diuretic (e.g., Furosemide 20–40 mg) in Patients with Normal or Mild Renal Impairment

Diuretics are used to increase potassium excretion in states of volume expansion such as heart failure. Furosemide can be started at a dose of 40–80 mg IV twice a day, but higher doses may be needed in renal impairment. For patients who are not hypervolemic, loop diuretics can be given with an infusion of IV saline to maintain euvolemia and urine flow with distal sodium delivery. Oral loop diuretics can be effective at lowering potassium levels in chronic renal failure.

Order a Low Potassium Diet

In patients with normal renal function, increased intake of potassium is generally well tolerated and is not a cause of hyperkalemia unless potassium is ingested in large quantities (>160 mEq) and is given as an IV bolus or if excretion of potassium is impaired. Still, it is important to take a dietary history to assess for high potassium intake that may be contributing to the persistence of hyperkalemia. Dietary sources of high potassium include tomatoes, white potatoes, sweet potatoes, bananas, oranges/orange juice, raisins, and salt substitutes. Restrict potassium in the diet to no more than 2 g per day.

Discontinue Any Medications That Impair Renal Potassium Excretion

Regardless of the urgency of potassium-lowering therapy, any medications that can cause hyperkalemia should be stopped or at least held temporarily. Angiotensin-converting enzyme inhibitors, angiotensin II receptor blockers, and aldosterone receptor blockers should be stopped. Other medications that can cause hyperkalemia include potassium-sparing diuretics, heparin, NSAIDs, calcineurin inhibitors, sulfamethoxazole/trimethoprim (Bactrim), and beta receptor antagonists. Depending on the severity and etiology of hyperkalemia, consider holding these medications as well.

Order Oral Sodium Polystyrene Sulfonate (Kayexalate) 15–30 g One to Four Times per Day in Non-postoperative Patients

Gastrointestinal cation exchangers remove potassium via exchange with other cations. Sodium polystyrene sulfonate removes potassium via exchange with sodium. It can be given as a single 15–30 g dose and repeated up to four times per day. The onset of action is at least 2 h and the maximum effect may take 6 or more hours. There is a small risk of intestinal necrosis with sodium polystyrene sulfonate, particularly in patients with underlying bowel disease and a bowel obstruction or who are postoperative, and therefore the safety of sodium polystyrene sulfonate has been widely debated. Many advocate for its use only with life-threatening hyperkalemia when dialysis is not readily available, while others use it routinely for control of hyperkalemia in CKD in the outpatient setting. With the development of newer cation exchangers including patiromer and zirconium cyclosilicate, sodium polystyrene sulfonate use is decreasing.

Obtain Nephrology Consultation for Hemodialysis in the Setting of ESRD, Advanced Renal Failure, or Patients with Rising Potassium Levels Not Responsive to Medical Therapy

End-stage renal disease patients presenting with hyperkalemia usually need urgent hemodialysis. These patients often tolerate higher serum levels of potassium, but renal consultation should be ordered immediately to assist with the timing of dialysis. Gastrointestinal cation exchangers are often recommended if hemodialysis cannot be performed immediately. Patients with oliguric or anuric acute renal failure will also need hemodialysis as loop diuretics are often not effective at promoting urinary potassium excretion. Temporizing measures described previously should be given while awaiting recommendations.

Fludrocortisone May Be Used in Patients With Aldosterone Deficiency

With demonstrated deficient aldosterone production, fludrocortisone can be used to correct the hyperkalemia. Start with an oral dose of 0.1 mg per day. Monitor for sodium retention, edema, and hypertension. Doses of up to 0.4 mg per day may be needed, particularly in cases of hyporeninemic hypoaldosteronism.

Suggested Reading

Kovesdy CP. Management of hyperkalemia: an update for the internist. Am J Med. 2015;128(12):1281–7.

Rose DB, Post DW. Hyperkalemia. In: Wonsciewicz M, McCullough K, Davis K, editors. Clinical physiology of acid-base and electrolyte disorders. 5th ed. New York: Mc-Graw Hill; 2001.

Sterns RH, Grieff M, Bernstein PL. Treatment of hyperkalemia: something old, something new. Kidney Int. 2016;89(3):546–54.

Weir MR, Rolfe M. Potassium homeostasis and renin-angiotensin-aldosterone system inhibitors. Treatment of hyperkalemia: something old, something new. Clin J Am Soc Nephrol. 2010;5(3):531–48.

Suspected Adrenocortical Deficiency

17

Anand Vaidya

Contents

A. Vaidya (✉)
Harvard Medical School, Center for Adrenal Disorders, Division
of Endocrinology, Diabetes, and Hypertension, Brigham and Women's
Hospital, Boston, MA, USA
e-mail: anandvaidya@bwh.harvard.edu

© Springer Nature Switzerland AG 2020
R. K. Garg et al. (eds.), *Handbook of Inpatient Endocrinology*,
https://doi.org/10.1007/978-3-030-38976-5_17

199

Physiological Considerations

The adrenal cortex synthesizes glucocorticoids and mineralocorticoids that physiologically regulate the acute response to stress, glycemic homeostasis, hemodynamic homeostasis, potassium and acid balance, immune function, organogenesis, parturition, and many other functions.

Adult adrenal glands are approximately 4 g in weight and usually 4 cm long and 2 cm wide and 1 cm thick lying on top of the superior pole of each kidney. On cross-sectional imaging (such as CT or MRI), they appear as thin and wispy structures that resemble a Mercedes-Benz symbol.

The adrenal gland is divided into the cortex and the medulla:

Cortex stems from mesenchymal tissue and synthesizes steroids. There are three histologic layers: zona glomerulosa (ZG) produces aldosterone, zona fasciculata (ZF) produces cortisol, and zona reticularis (ZR) produces DHEA and androstenedione.

Medulla, which is the core of the adrenal, arises from neural crest cells and functions primarily to synthesize catecholamines.

The regulation of cortisol and androgen synthesis is entirely dependent on ACTH. Aldosterone synthesis is also stimulated by ACTH; however, the synthesis of aldosterone is also potently stimulated by angiotensin II (thus activation of the renin-angiotensin system stimulates adrenal aldosterone) and by high extracellular potassium. Therefore, in contrast to cortisol synthesis, aldosterone synthesis is not dependent on ACTH. Adrenal androgens play a minor role in adult human physiology but are important for adrenarche, including the development of axillary and pubic hair. Cortisol is a glucocorticoid that binds to and activates the glucocorticoid receptor (GR), but it is also a mineralocorticoid that can potently activate the mineralocorticoid receptor (MR). Cortisol is the main glucocorticoid in human physiology and therefore is the dominant ligand for the GR. Activation of the GR raises blood glucose, increases blood pressure, suppresses immune activity/inflammation, increases appetite, and depresses mood. These physiologic actions explain the pathophysiologic manifestations of diseases with cortisol deficiency (adrenal insufficiency) and cortisol excess (Cushing syndrome).

Aldosterone is a pure mineralocorticoid and only activates the MR, principally in the distal nephron but also in other tissues such as the colon, heart, and vasculature. Activation of the renal MR increases renal sodium reabsorption, which facilitates the retention of water and results in intravascular volume expansion. Activation of the renal MR also increases renal potassium and hydrogen ion excretion. Therefore, another key role of aldosterone is to ensure normal potassium homeostasis and acid-base status by regulating urinary potassium and proton excretion. Notably, cortisol is also a potent mineralocorticoid and can activate the MR. Although cortisol circulates in the blood in 100- to 1000-fold higher concentrations than aldosterone, MR over-activation (such as in primary aldosteronism) resulting in sodium retention, volume expansion, high blood pressure, and hypokalemia is prevented by 11β-hydroxysteroid dehydrogenase type 2 (11βHSD2), which is co-expressed with the MR in the kidney, and functions to convert cortisol to the inactive cortisone. In this manner, 11βHSD2 inactivates the majority of cortisol before it can bind to and activate the renal MR.

The classical control of the adrenal cortex involves communications between the hypothalamus, pituitary, and adrenal. The hypothalamus secretes corticotropin-releasing hormone (CRH), which stimulates the secretion of ACTH from the corticotrophs of the anterior pituitary. Cortisol binds to peripheral GR but also the centrally expressed GR in the hypothalamus and pituitary. Therefore, cortisol negatively regulates CRH and ACTH.

ACTH also stimulates aldosterone secretion from the adrenal cortex; however, the dominant secretagogues of aldosterone are angiotensin II and potassium. Therefore, the predominant axis that regulates aldosterone is the renin-angiotensin system.

Aldosterone acts on the MR expressed in the distal nephron to increase sodium retention and thereby expand the intravascular volume to counter the initial insult of renal hypoperfusion. This closes the renin-angiotensin-aldosterone feedback loop. High extracellular potassium also stimulates adrenal aldosterone production, and in turn activation of the MR by aldosterone increases urinary potassium excretion in the distal nephron to close this feedback loop.

One of the major roles of cortisol is to help the body defend against stress. Stress can be defined as any physical or emotional stress or any condition that is perceived to be a threat or fear. In this regard, the stress response is designed to permit physiologic changes that defend against stress. The perception of stress stimulates CRH via central nervous system inputs. Other stressors such as hypoglycemia, hypotension, pain, and fever all stimulate the hypothalamic release of CRH to activate the axis and result in increases in cortisol *proportional to the degree of stress* to counter these stimuli. Vasopressin (also called antidiuretic hormone [ADH]), can stimulate pituitary ACTH secretion, as can cytokines that are increased during infections or inflammatory conditions.

Another major regulator of the hypothalamic-pituitary-adrenal axis is light, thus creating a circadian rhythm. From a diagnostic standpoint, this diurnal secretion of cortisol is one of the main reasons why the diagnosis of adrenal insufficiency can be challenging.

What Is a Normal Cortisol Level?

A robust and elevated peak morning cortisol suggests a normal functioning hypothalamic-pituitary-adrenal axis; however, determining when that peak arises and should be measured is often the challenge, particularly in the inpatient setting. Specific thresholds will be discussed below in Diagnosis.

Primary and Secondary Adrenal Insufficiencies

The term adrenal insufficiency refers to an *absolute or* relative deficiency of adrenal cortical hormones (cortisol and/or aldosterone) with respect to the current needs of the body.

Primary Adrenal Insufficiency

Primary adrenal insufficiency (Addison's disease) refers to the destruction or inhibition of the entire adrenal cortex, resulting in an inability to synthesize and secrete cortisol and aldosterone (as well as androgens). The main signs and symptoms of this condition are due to the lack of cortisol and aldosterone. In the absence of negative feedback from cortisol, the hypothalamus and pituitary augment secretion of CRH, POMC, and as a result ACTH and melanocyte-stimulating hormone (MSH).

Secondary Adrenal Insufficiency

Secondary adrenal insufficiency refers to the destruction or inhibition of the corticotroph cells in the anterior pituitary. Secretion of ACTH will be relatively insufficient or completely deficient. In the absence of ACTH, the adrenal cortex is not stimulated, and adrenal steroidogenesis is inhibited. This is particularly evident for cortisol and androgens. Since aldosterone synthesis and secretion can continue to be stimulated by angiotensin II and potassium, secondary adrenal insufficiency is mainly a syndrome of cortisol insufficiency; aldosterone regulation continues unabated.

Clinical Presentation and Diagnosis

Primary Adrenal Insufficiency

Primary adrenal insufficiency typically presents with marked or critical illness. General malaise and feelings of being unwell, gastrointestinal symptoms (nausea, vomiting, diarrhea, abdominal pain), and, in severe circumstances, hypoglycemia and hypotension are hallmarks of the illness and may be ongoing and progressively worsening for months to years before the diagnosis is made. Aldosterone insufficiency makes these patients especially vulnerable. In the absence of aldosterone, renal sodium reabsorption is not maximal, resulting in renal sodium wasting and progressive intravascular volume depletion. This can manifest as symptoms of lightheadedness and orthostasis (dizziness and lightheadedness upon standing from a seated position) and frankly low blood pressure (hypotension and circulatory collapse) and salt cravings. Diffuse hyperpigmentation of the skin, particularly marked surrounding scar tissue and on mucosal membranes (such as the buccal mucosa and vaginal mucosa), is attributed to the high circulating levels of MSH- and ACTH-stimulating melanocytes. Primary adrenal insufficiency can be diagnosed by simultaneously evaluating a cortisol and ACTH – a relatively low or frankly low cortisol levels and concomitantly marked elevations in ACTH. Morning cortisol levels less than 5 mcg/dL confirm the diagnosis of adrenal insufficiency, along with a concomitant ACTH level that is at least twofold greater than the upper range of normal (but usually several hundred or even greater than a thousand, pg/mL). Further, the deficiency of aldosterone may result in hyponatremia, hyperkalemia, and a markedly elevated renin. Measuring a renin and aldosterone is recommended to assess the degree of mineralocorticoid deficiency in primary adrenal insufficiency. Patients with primary adrenal insufficiency will exhibit low serum aldosterone levels, despite low blood pressure and high potassium balance, and markedly elevated plasma renin activity. Performing a cosyntropin stimulation (measuring a morning cortisol level, then injecting 250 mcg of synthetic ACTH-like peptide, followed by repeat cortisol measure at 30 and 60 min) can further confirm the diagnosis. Because the pathophysiology involves destruction of the adrenal cortex, patients with primary adrenal insufficiency disease exhibit markedly diminished cortisol stimulation when cosyntropin is injected. A failure to achieve a peak stimulated cortisol following cosyntropin of > 18 mcg/dL indicates adrenal insufficiency.

Secondary Adrenal Insufficiency

Secondary adrenal insufficiency can present with a wide variety of signs and symptoms. This is in part because aldosterone regulation is intact and therefore hemodynamic homeostasis may be intact. The clinical syndrome experienced by these patients reflects the degree of stress (physical or emotional) they are under and the disparity between how much cortisol they are able to produce and how much cortisol is needed at any given time. For example, a healthy patient with secondary adrenal insufficiency and a relatively low cortisol may experience no symptoms or perhaps only mild weakness and fatigue. However, as the degree of stress the patient experiences increases (e.g., the development of a febrile illness like influenza or sustaining severe trauma and pain), the gap between the patient's need for cortisol and ability to produce cortisol increases, and the clinical manifestations become more severe. Ultimately, in the setting of severe stress or critical illness, these patients may develop a clinical syndrome that includes intravascular volume depletion and hypotension, resembling that of primary adrenal insufficiency. Secondary adrenal insufficiency is diagnosed by confirming an inappropriately low morning cortisol level (ideally < 5 mcg/dL) in combination with an inappropriately low ACTH. A suboptimal cosyntropin stimulation test (peak cortisol < 18 mcg/dL) can provide further confirmation of the diagnosis of adrenal insufficiency and insight into the chronicity of the problem. A robust and normal peak cortisol following cosyntropin indicates that the lack of ACTH is acute or subacute (hours, days, or a few weeks). A suboptimal response to cosyntropin suggests that the deficiency of ACTH is chronic (weeks to months); since ACTH is trophic to the adrenal cortex, prolonged deficiency results in atrophy of the zona fasciculata and progressively diminished responses to cosyntropin.

Adrenal Insufficiency in Critically Ill Patients

Adrenal insufficiency in critically ill patients is often more challenging to diagnose than in noncritically ill patients because critically ill patients (1) may not have normal circadian rhythms, (2) may have decreased metabolism and clearance of cortisol, and (3) may have reduced circulating binding globulins, thus lowering total cortisol but not necessarily free and bioavailable cortisol.

An important response to critical illness is a rise in ACTH. Whereas some hypothalamic and pituitary hormones may exhibit a physiological suppression during critical illness, critical illness should result in a robust rise in ACTH and increased adrenal cortical stimulation. Therefore, theoretically, patients with critical illness should have appropriately elevated cortisol levels, in part because ACTH is elevated and also because cortisol metabolism is decreased. In patients who have markedly reduced concentrations of albumin, cortisol-binding globulin may also be decreased and, therefore, total cortisol levels may decline and correlation with presumed free cortisol levels may become more challenging. Measuring cortisol-binding globulin or free cortisol levels may be useful. However, because these assays are not routinely performed and may take days to weeks to return, they are not commonly used in the practical diagnosis and management of adrenal insufficiency. Rather, it is generally suggested that a critically ill patient with a relatively normal albumin of >2.5 g/dL and cortisol of <15 mcg/dL is indicative of adrenal insufficiency that may require glucocorticoid replacement therapy. In contrast, in a critically ill patient with more marked hypoalbuminemia (albumin <2.5 g/dL), a random cortisol of <10 mcg/dL may indicate adrenal insufficiency. When a critically ill patient is hypotensive due to septic shock and resistant to vasopressor therapy, empiric treatment with glucocorticoids without diagnostic testing may be considered as an emergency measure.

Etiology

Primary adrenal insufficiency, particularly in developed parts of the world, is most commonly autoimmune adrenalitis. It may occur in isolation, or as a part of a larger autoimmune polyglandular syndrome. Other causes of primary adrenal insufficiency include bilateral infiltrative infections (such as tuberculosis and fungi), bilateral adrenal hemorrhage, infiltrative malignancies, bilateral adrenalectomy, congenital adrenal hyperplasia, adrenoleukodystrophy, and rarer genetic syndromes. Establishing the cause of primary adrenal insufficiency is important. A positive 21-hydroxylase antibody can provide reassurance for autoimmune adrenalitis, whereas when the titer is negative, evaluation for other causes using serologic testing and/or imaging should be considered. The evaluation of other non-autoimmune causes should be considered on a case-by-case basis depending on the practice location and pretest probability. Imaging of the adrenals can help identify hemorrhage, infiltrative infections, and malignancy. Suspicion for adrenoleukodystrophy can be confirmed with imaging and assessment of very long chain fatty acids. Evaluation for congenital adrenal hyper- or hypoplasia is best performed by measuring intermediate adrenal steroids. Certain medications can inhibit adrenal steroidogenesis transiently and result in a functional primary adrenal insufficiency: antifungal medications, etomidate, and, rarely, heparin.

Secondary adrenal insufficiency can be the result of any condition that interrupts or damages the hypothalamus and pituitary. These include principally benign pituitary or parasellar tumors and rarely primary or metastatic brain malignancy, infection, hemorrhage, infiltrative diseases, and radiation that involved the hypothalamus or pituitary. The most common cause of secondary adrenal insufficiency, however, is iatrogenic secondary adrenal insufficiency due to the frequent use of exogenous glucocorticoids (most often oral or intravenous but in some instances inhaled and topical as well). Opioid medications are also frequently used and in some instances can cause a transient suppression of ACTH.

Treatment

Primary Adrenal Insufficiency

The treatment of primary adrenal insufficiency is focused on replacing the missing vital adrenal steroids: cortisol and aldosterone. Patients are typically treated with a glucocorticoid (such as hydrocortisone or prednisone) and in addition with a mineralocorticoid (such as fludrocortisone) to replace their deficiencies (Table 17.1). The choice of glucocorticoid can vary, but the most preferred option in adults is hydrocortisone (15–25 mg daily) in two divided doses, often the larger dose first thing in the morning and the smaller dose in the early afternoon. Hydrocortisone peaks within 1–3 h and nadirs within 5–7 h, thus providing an opportunity to give a physiologic regimen of glucocorticoid. A common glucocorticoid regimen is hydrocortisone 15–20 mg upon awakening and 10 mg between 12 and 2 pm. Some patients require a third smaller dose in the early evening. Prednisolone (3–5 mg daily) and prednisone (5–7.5 mg daily) are alternatives that can be given once or twice daily but have longer half-lives and therefore less physiologic profiles. Dexamethasone is not ideal since it has a very long half-life and the greatest risk for inducing Cushingoid effects. Efficacy of glucocorticoid dosing is determined by patient well-being, energy level, normal blood pressure, and electrolytes. Toxicity or signs of excessive glucocorticoid dosing are determined by evidence of weight gain and other Cushingoid signs. All patients with mineralocorticoid deficiency should be treated with fludrocortisone, typically 0.05–0.15 mg once daily. The efficacy of fludrocortisone dosing can be monitored by observing normal blood pressure (without postural hypotension), normal sodium and potassium balance, and the lowering of the previously elevated renin levels. Patients should be instructed on how to remain well hydrated and consume sufficient dietary sodium, especially on warmer days when insensible loses of water and salt can be greater.

Table 17.1 Treatment of primary adrenal insufficiency

	Maintenance	Minor-moderate illness	Moderate-severe illness or surgery
Formulation/dose/action	Glucocorticoid: hydrocortisone 15–25 mg in two divided doses; alternatively prednisolone 3–5 mg daily or prednisone 5–7.5 mg daily Mineralocorticoid: fludrocortisone 0.05–0.15 mg in a single dose	Double (fever >38 °C) or triple (fever >39 °C) glucocorticoid dose for 2–3 days, increase hydration with water and electrolyte-rich fluids	If emesis and inability to take oral medications or fluids: intramuscular or intravenous hydrocortisone 50–100 mg and intravenous fluids If major surgery with general anesthesia, intensive care hospitalization, or delivery: 50–100 mg of intravenous hydrocortisone every 6–8 h and intravenous fluids If adrenal crisis: aggressive hydration with isotonic fluids, hydrocortisone 100 mg intravenous every 4–6 h
Typical example	Hydrocortisone 15–20 mg in the morning and 5–10 mg in the early afternoon *and* fludrocortisone 0.10 mg in the morning	Double hydrocortisone dose for 2–3 days until mild febrile illness abates	Intravenous hydrocortisone 50–100 mg Intramuscular hydrocortisone 100 mg

(continued)

Table 17.1 (continued)

	Maintenance	Minor-moderate illness	Moderate-severe illness or surgery
Comment	The dose of glucocorticoid and mineralocorticoid can vary depending on the size of the patient, daily activity and workload (physical or other), and other symptoms. During exercise, additional or higher doses may be required. A general rule of thumb to minimize supraphysiologic glucocorticoid effects is to establish the lowest dose of glucocorticoid that enables a good quality of life	If symptoms do not abate or worsen, in-person evaluation should be conducted	In addition to higher glucocorticoid dosing, hydration with isotonic fluids is a critical management element. For patients unable to maintain oral hydration, intravenous hydration with isotonic fluids should be initiated

Secondary Adrenal Insufficiency

The treatment of secondary adrenal insufficiency is focused on replacing glucocorticoids. Patients are typically treated with hydrocortisone or prednisone (Table 17.2). If the cause of secondary adrenal insufficiency was iatrogenic glucocorticoid administration, then the goal of therapy should be to gradually taper the glucocorticoid down in hopes that the endogenous hypothalamic-pituitary-adrenal axis will revive and resume normal function. The precise tapering schedule can vary and should be created on a case-by-case basis and customized for the specific patient. The longer the exposure to supraphysiologic glucocorticoids, the more profound the inhibition of endogenous ACTH production and the longer the time to recovery. Symptoms of fatigue, orthostasis, and/or depression may be signs that they are experiencing relative

Table 17.2 Treatment of secondary adrenal insufficiencies

	Maintenance	Minor-moderate illness	Moderate-severe illness or surgery
Formulation/ dose/action	Glucocorticoid: hydrocortisone 10–25 mg in two divided doses; alternatively prednisolone 1–5 mg daily or prednisone 3–7.5 mg daily Mineralocorticoid: none	Double (fever >38 °C) or triple (fever >39 °C) glucocorticoid dose for 2–3 days, increase hydration with water and electrolyte-rich fluids	If emesis and inability to take oral medications or fluids: intramuscular or intravenous hydrocortisone 50–100 mg and intravenous fluids If major surgery with general anesthesia, intensive care hospitalization, or delivery: 50–100 mg of intravenous hydrocortisone every 6–8 h and intravenous fluids If adrenal crisis: aggressive hydration with isotonic fluids, hydrocortisone 100 mg intravenous every 4–6 h
Typical example	Hydrocortisone 10–20 mg in the morning and 5–10 mg in the early afternoon *or* prednisone 3–7.5 mg in the morning	Double hydrocortisone or prednisone dose for 2–3 days until mild febrile illness abates	Intravenous hydrocortisone 50–100 mg Intramuscular hydrocortisone 100 mg

(continued)

Table 17.2 (continued)

	Maintenance	Minor-moderate illness	Moderate-severe illness or surgery
Comment	The dose of glucocorticoid can vary depending on the size of the patient, daily activity and workload (physical or other), and other symptoms. During exercise, additional or higher doses may be required. A general rule of thumb to minimize supraphysiologic glucocorticoid effects is to establish the lowest dose of glucocorticoid that enables a good quality of life. If the cause of secondary adrenal insufficiency was iatrogenic glucocorticoid administration, then the goal of therapy should be to gradually taper the glucocorticoid doses to permit normalization of the hypothalamic-pituitary-adrenal axis. The precise tapering schedule can vary and should be created on a case-by-case basis and customized for the specific patient. The longer the exposure to supraphysiologic glucocorticoids, the more profound the inhibition of endogenous ACTH production and the longer the time to recovery	If symptoms do not abate or worsen, in-person evaluation should be conducted	In addition to higher glucocorticoid dosing, hydration with isotonic fluids is a critical management element. For patients unable to maintain oral hydration, intravenous hydration with isotonic fluids should be initiated

adrenal insufficiency and should prompt consideration to slow the pace of the taper. Measuring a morning cortisol and ACTH, 24 h after the last dose of glucocorticoid, can provide insight into the status of the hypothalamic-pituitary-adrenal axis. Low levels of each suggest a profound suppression of the axis. A rise in ACTH with a low cortisol suggests an awakening of the pituitary corticotrophs and stimulation of the zona fasciculata by supraphysiologic ACTH, following which a gradual rise in cortisol should following the subsequent weeks to months. A morning cortisol greater than 10 mcg/dL, but ideally >15–18 mcg/dL, indicates restoration of normal endogenous HPA axis function and a concomitant completion of the glucocorticoid taper. In addition, serial cosyntropin stimulation tests can be performed during the taper to evaluate not only basal ACTH and cortisol levels but also the magnitude of the stimulated value, to either assess normalization of adrenal function or provide data to estimate the progress and duration of the glucocorticoid taper. Most patients with secondary adrenal insufficiency do not need mineralocorticoid replacement.

Stress Dosing

Stress dosing of glucocorticoids is important counseling that should be provided to all patients with adrenal insufficiency. During critical illness, febrile illness, trauma, and/or other physical stressors, the glucocorticoid needs of the body may increase. Patients reliant on exogenous glucocorticoids must therefore anticipate this by increasing their oral glucocorticoid dosing. Patients should typically be advised to double or triple their glucocorticoid doses during these situations, for a duration of a few days. If the illness and increased glucocorticoid dosing extends beyond 2–3 days, patients should seek counsel from their physicians to determine the necessity of glucocorticoid increases and search for potential causes of the illness. Gastrointestinal illnesses are notoriously the most concerning. Viral gastroenteritis inducing vomiting or diarrhea can result in volume depletion and lack of absorption (or intake) of steroids. Patients with adrenal insufficiency can quickly spiral into a hemodynamic crisis in these situations and should be instructed to either go to an emergency room for intravenous hydration and steroid injections or be capable of self-injecting intramuscular hydrocortisone or dexamethasone. Patients with primary adrenal insufficiency are more susceptible to adrenal crisis with gastrointestinal illness given their mineralocorticoid deficiency. Patients should all be advised to wear a medic-alert bracelet or necklace that indicates that they have adrenal insufficiency for emergency providers. It is generally advisable to prescribe for them intramuscular hydrocortisone (100 mg) or dexamethasone in case they are not in proximity of an emergency room during an adrenal crisis.

Suggested Reading

Boonen E, Vervenne H, Meersseman P, Andrew R, Mortier L, Declercq PE, et al. Reduced cortisol metabolism during critical illness. N Engl J Med. 2013;368(16):1477–88.

Bornstein SR, Allolio B, Arlt W, Barthel A, Don-Wauchope A, Hammer GD, et al. Diagnosis and treatment of primary adrenal insufficiency: an endocrine society clinical practice guideline. J Clin Endocrinol Metab. 2016;101(2):364–89.

Gomez-Sanchez CE. Adrenal dysfunction in critically ill patients. N Engl J Med. 2013;368(16):1547–9.

Guran T, Buonocore F, Saka N, Ozbek MN, Aycan Z, Bereket A, et al. Rare causes of primary adrenal insufficiency: genetic and clinical characterization of a large nationwide cohort. J Clin Endocrinol Metab. 2016;101(1):284–92.

Hamrahian AH, Fleseriu M, AACE Adrenal Scientific Committee. Evaluation and management of adrenal insufficiency in critically ill patients: disease state review. Endocr Pract. 2017;23(6):716–25.

Cushing's Syndrome

18

Brandon P. Galm and Nicholas A. Tritos

Contents

B. P. Galm (✉)
Neuroendocrine Unit, Massachusetts General Hospital and Harvard
Medical School, Boston, MA, USA

N. A. Tritos
Harvard Medical School, Massachusetts General Hospital,
Neuroendocrine Unit and Neuroendocrine & Pituitary Tumor Clinical
Center, Boston, MA, USA
e-mail: ntritos@mgh.harvard.edu

© Springer Nature Switzerland AG 2020
R. K. Garg et al. (eds.), *Handbook of Inpatient Endocrinology*,
https://doi.org/10.1007/978-3-030-38976-5_18

Consider Testing for Cushing's Syndrome if the Patient Has a Cluster of Suggestive Signs and Symptoms, Unusual Symptoms or Features for Age (e.g., Hypertension or Osteoporosis in a Younger Patient), a Pituitary Gland Mass, or an Adrenal Adenoma

Consider testing for Cushing's syndrome (CS) in the setting of a cluster of suggestive signs or symptoms (Table 18.1), although many are nonspecific when present in isolation, and in the setting of unusual symptoms or features for the patient's age, such as unexplained hypertension or osteoporosis in a younger patient. The most discriminative (specific but not sensitive) features are reddish/purple striae > 1 cm wide, proximal

Table 18.1 Features of Cushing's syndrome

Metabolic	Cardiovascular	Catabolic
Central adiposity	Hypertension	Proximal
Hyperglycemia/diabetes	Myocardial infarction	myopathy
Hypertension	Cardiomyopathy	Bone loss
Hypertriglyceridemia	Stroke	Striae
Facial plethora	Venous	Ecchymoses
Fat redistribution (dorsal fat	thromboembolism	Skin thinning
pad, supraclavicular fullness,		Weight loss
facial fullness)		
Hypogonadal	Mineralocorticoid	Hyperandrogenic (women)
Reduced fertility	Hypokalemia	Acne
Low libido	Metabolic alkalosis	Hirsutism
Irregular menses	Hypertension	Oligomenorrhea
	Edema	
Neuropsychiatric	Others	Pediatric
Depression, anxiety	Nephrolithiasis	Decreased growth
Emotional lability	Infections	velocity
Mania	Exophthalmos	Altered timing of
Changes in cognition	Avascular necrosis	puberty
Lethargy	Skin	
Insomnia	hyperpigmentation	
Psychosis	(ACTH-dependent)	

myopathy, facial plethora, spontaneous ecchymoses, and disproportionate, central adiposity. Some patients, especially those with biochemically severe ectopic CS, may present in a catabolic state, with weight loss, muscle wasting, edema, and severe hypokalemia. In addition, consider testing for CS if the patient has an incidental pituitary gland lesion suggestive of an adenoma. Most guidelines recommend that patients with an incidental adrenal lesion consistent with an adenoma should undergo testing for CS, usually with the low-dose 1-mg dexamethasone suppression test (DST).

Use of Exogenous Glucocorticoids Is the Most Common Cause of Cushing's Syndrome in the General Population and Should Always Be Considered First in the Evaluation of Patients with Suspected Hypercortisolism

The use of exogenous glucocorticoids is the most common cause of CS. This includes any route of administration, such as topical, inhaled, intra-articular, and rectal. Make sure to ask about joint injections (including the spine) over the last few months. Make sure to ask about strong cytochrome P450 (CYP450) inhibitors, especially ritonavir or cobicistat (antiretroviral therapy), as these increase the risk of CS with exogenous steroid use. Also ask about naturopathic or herbal supplements. Megestrol acetate (Megace®), an appetite stimulant, has glucocorticoid activity and can cause CS. Patients on exogenous steroids may appear Cushingoid with biochemical evidence of hypoadrenalism as a result of suppression of the pituitary-adrenal axis, including a low or undetectable serum cortisol level (if the exogenous glucocorticoid has limited cross-reactivity with cortisol in the assay) and low plasma ACTH. Exogenous glucocorticoids may be detectable in urine specimens assayed by liquid chromatography tandem mass spectrometry, though this test is rarely needed in clinical practice.

Endogenous Cushing's Syndrome Can Be Caused by Lesions of the Pituitary Gland ("Cushing's Disease"), Adrenal Glands, or Other Organs (Ectopic ACTH-Secreting Tumors)

Causes of endogenous CS are shown in Table 18.2.

Table 18.2 Causes of endogenous Cushing's syndrome

ACTH-dependent	Pituitary (70%)	Pituitary adenoma (Cushing's disease; CD)	Females 3–5 times more, peak 20–30s, 95% are microadenomas
	Ectopic ACTH[a] (10%)	Small cell lung cancer	Peak 40–50s, especially smokers
		Carcinoids (bronchial, thymic)	Peak 20–30s
		Others[b]	Rare, may have other paraneoplastic syndromes
ACTH-independent	Adrenal (20%)	Adrenal adenoma (60%)	Females 4–8 times more, peak 30–40s
		Adrenal carcinoma (40%)	Females 1–3 times more, peak 40–50s, often large mass, may co-secrete androgens
		Bilateral nodular adrenal hyperplasia[c] (<1%)	May be familial or associated with Carney complex

[a]May rarely be caused by ectopic CRH secretion (<1% of ACTH-dependent CS)
[b]Includes pancreatic neuroendocrine tumors, pheochromocytoma, medullary thyroid carcinoma, and others
[c]Includes bilateral macronodular adrenal hyperplasia and primary pigmented nodular adrenocortical disease

Diagnostic Testing Should Be Optimally Deferred to the Outpatient Setting Unless the Patient Has Acute Manifestations or Severe Comorbidities Potentially Related to Hypercortisolism

Defer testing for CS to the outpatient setting, if possible (e.g., incidental adrenal or pituitary adenoma), as many tests may be difficult to interpret in the hospitalized patient and may not have been adequately validated in this population. Physiologic hypercortisolism (pseudo-Cushing's syndrome) can be seen in severe obesity and in acute stress and illness, including depression, poorly controlled diabetes mellitus, and malnutrition, and 50–80% will have abnormal testing for CS. However, it is important to remember that patients with acute manifestations or severe comorbidities (such as sepsis, psychosis, or severe, unexplained hypokalemia with cachexia) that are suspected of being hypercortisolemic require urgent evaluation and management in the inpatient setting.

Confirm Pathologic, Autonomous Hypercortisolism as the First Step

Order the 24-h urinary free cortisol (UFC) (at least two collections), late-night salivary cortisol (LNSC) (at least two samples), and/or the low-dose 1-mg DST. Urine creatinine and volume should be measured with UFC tests to ensure adequate collection and exclude high urinary volumes as an explanation for falsely elevated UFC. Consider measuring a plasma dexamethasone level during the DST to ensure adequate exposure during the test. The 2-day DST is usually deferred to the outpatient setting. At least two different tests should be positive before pathologic hypercortisolism is confirmed. Significant fluctuations of cortisol secretion can be seen, especially in the setting of cyclic CS. LNSC is rarely done in hospital due to the delayed turnaround time. Test characteristics are shown in Table 18.3.

Table 18.3 Initial tests used to evaluate for pathologic hypercortisolism (Cushing's syndrome)

Test	Cutoff	Sensitivity	Specificity	False positives	False negatives
1 mg DST	>1.8 μg/dL	97–100%	80–90%	Estrogens (OCP), CYP inducers[a], rapid metabolizers	CYP inhibitors[b]
UFC	>ULN[c]	80–95%	90–95%	Fluid intake >5 L/day, some drugs[d]	Reduced GFR
LNSC	>ULN[c]	90–95%	95–100%	Tobacco or licorice use, altered sleep-wakefulness cycle	

Abbreviations: CYP cytochrome P450, *DST* dexamethasone suppression test, *GFR* glomerular filtration rate, *LNSC* late-night salivary cortisol, *OCP* oral contraceptive pill, *UFC* 24-h urinary free cortisol, *ULN* upper limit of normal
[a]Strong CYP450 inducers include phenytoin, carbamazepine, rifampin, phenobarbital, ethosuximide, and pioglitazone
[b]Strong CYP450 inhibitors include azole antifungals, ritonavir, fluoxetine, diltiazem, and cimetidine
[c]Use the reference range provided by the laboratory, as assay types and cutoffs vary. Specificity for CS rises with greater UFC or LNSC elevations; however, the effects of acute illness on cortisol levels should also be considered when interpreting test results
[d]Carbamazepine, fenofibrate (in some assays), licorice, and carbenoxolone

Measure Plasma ACTH to Direct Further Investigations

Once CS is confirmed, measure plasma ACTH to determine whether CS is ACTH-dependent or ACTH-independent. ACTH is optimally assayed in morning specimens. Ensure that ACTH is collected properly, as it is degraded quickly and needs to be placed on ice immediately after collection. CS is ACTH-dependent if ACTH is inappropriately normal or high (>20 pg/mL), while it is ACTH-independent if ACTH is suppressed (<5 pg/mL) in a patient with active hypercortisolism. Intermediate levels (5–20 pg/mL) may represent either possibility but are more often ACTH-dependent.

Order a Pituitary-Directed MRI in ACTH-Dependent Cushing's Syndrome

Order a pituitary-directed MRI to investigate for a pituitary adenoma, although this may miss 40–50% of small adenomas causing CS. Recall that pituitary incidentalomas occur in ~10% of the general population. Unless there is an adenoma >6–10 mm, proceed with inferior petrosal sinus sampling (IPSS) to distinguish pituitary from ectopic CS. The high-dose DST is also sometimes used but has low specificity (~67%), and results should generally be confirmed on IPSS. For ectopic CS, order CT of the chest, abdomen, and pelvis. If this does not identify a source, functional nuclear imaging (octreotide scan, FDG PET, F-DOPA PET, or gallium DOTATATE PET) may be required.

Order Adrenal Imaging in ACTH-Independent Cushing's Syndrome

Order adrenal imaging (CT or MRI) to investigate for an adrenal mass. Recognize that adrenal incidentalomas occur in ~10% of the population but are more likely to be the source of CS when hypercortisolism is present and ACTH is suppressed. Patients with ACTH-independent CS and bilateral adrenal adenomatous lesions may require adrenal vein sampling to determine which lesion is the culprit. Also order adrenal androgens to assess for co-secretion, which is common in adrenal carcinomas; in contrast, serum DHEA-S is typically below normal in adrenal CS due to adrenal adenomas.

Assess and Manage Hypercortisolism-Related Consequences and Comorbidities

Assess for the presence of hyperglycemia, hypertension, dyslipidemia, and osteoporosis, and manage these as per usual. Assess for psychiatric disorders and consider referral to psychiatry if appropriate. Offer appropriate vaccinations, especially for pneumococcus, influenza, and (preferably not during active hypercortisolism) herpes zoster. Hypokalemia from overstimulation of the mineralocorticoid receptor by excess cortisol (especially in ectopic CS) should be monitored and treated with potassium supplements and spironolactone or eplerenone. Consider prophylaxis for venous thromboembolism, especially perioperatively and in those at high risk. Consider prophylaxis for opportunistic infections, especially *Pneumocystis*, in severe CS (UFC > 5 × ULN).

Refer for Tumor-Directed Surgery as First-Line Therapy for Cushing's Syndrome

When localization has been successful, surgery (transsphenoidal pituitary surgery, unilateral adrenalectomy, or resection of ectopic tumor) performed by an experienced surgeon is first-line therapy for those who are appropriate candidates. Control of hypercortisolism and its associated comorbidities, especially when severe, should be considered prior to surgery. If the source of CS cannot be identified (especially in ectopic CS), bilateral adrenalectomy may be an option, especially in life-threatening severe CS or in those who have contraindications or are refractory to medical therapy.

Consider Pharmacotherapy Prior to Surgery, if Surgery Is Contraindicated or Tumor Location Is Unknown, if the Patient Is Medically Unstable, or for Persistent or Recurrent Cushing's Syndrome After Surgery

Options for pharmacotherapy are shown in Table 18.4. For rapid control, patients are usually started on ketoconazole and/or metyrapone (mifepristone may also be considered, if available). For very rapid control in life-threatening CS in the critical care setting, etomidate may be useful but requires close monitoring for sedation. Cabergoline or pasireotide may be more useful in

Table 18.4 Pharmacotherapy for Cushing's syndrome

Medication	Mechanism of action	Approximate efficacy[a]	Dosing	Adverse effects
Cabergoline	Dopamine receptor 2 agonist	30–40%	1–7 mg/wk	GI upset, orthostatic hypotension, potentially cardiac valvulopathy in high doses
Pasireotide	Somatostatin receptor ligand	20–40%	600–1200 μg sc bid[c]	GI upset, cholelithiasis, transaminitis, hyperglycemia/diabetes, prolonged QT
Ketoconazole	Inhibits several adrenal enzymes	50–75%	400–1600 mg/d, divided bid–tid	Transaminitis, hepatitis, drug interactions, gynecomastia, hypogonadism (men)
Metyrapone	Inhibits 11β-hydroxylase	50–75%	500–6000 mg/d, divided tid–qid	GI upset, hirsutism, acne, hypokalemia, edema, hypertension
Etomidate	Inhibits several adrenal enzymes	100% (dose-dependent)	3–5 mg load then 0.03–0.1 mg/kg/h	Sedation; requires monitoring in intensive care, given via central line
Mitotane	Adrenolytic, inhibits several adrenal enzymes	75–85%	250–8000 mg/d, divided tid–qid	GI upset, CNS effects, transaminitis, alters binding proteins, inhibits CYP 3A4, drug interactions, hypothyroidism, teratogenic
Mifepristone	Glucocorticoid receptor antagonist	40–60%[b]	300–1200 mg once daily	GI upset, abortifacient, hypokalemia, hypertension, edema, endometrial thickening

Abbreviations: CNS central nervous system, *CYP* cytochrome P450, *GI* gastrointestinal

[a]All estimates are approximate, as various studies used different outcomes for efficacy. Treatment escape may develop in some patients (~25% on cabergoline, ~10% on ketoconazole, ~5% on metyrapone)

[b]As cortisol and UFC are not meaningful while on mifepristone, efficacy is reported as improvement in diabetes or hypertension

[c]A long-acting formulation of pasireotide (10–40 mg intramuscularly every 4 weeks) has also been tested and FDA-approved for the treatment of CS

less-severe pituitary CS but take longer to control hypercortisolism than adrenally acting agents. Combination therapy can also be useful (efficacious in 70–90%), especially in severe or refractory CS. Monitoring while hospitalized is generally performed with serum cortisol (although UFC can be used), with a target of ~10–15 µg/dL (exact targets vary depending on assay). Do not monitor cortisol levels in patients on mifepristone. All agents can cause hypoadrenalism as an extension of their pharmacologic effects. Only pasireotide and mifepristone are FDA-approved for treatment of CS.

Consider Pituitary Radiotherapy in Persistent or Recurrent Cushing's Disease or if Surgery Is Contraindicated

Consider pituitary-directed radiotherapy (RT) for refractory, persistent, or recurrent CD, for patients with contraindications to surgery, or for large adenomas with residual tumor after surgical debulking. As RT may take months to years to become effective, other medical therapies may need to be used in the interim.

Consider Bilateral Adrenalectomy in Patients Who Have Refractory Cushing's Syndrome

Consider bilateral adrenalectomy in patients who have refractory CS despite medical therapy, tumor-directed surgery, and/or RT. Bilateral adrenalectomy may also be helpful in severe, life-threatening CS and in patients where the primary tumor (including ectopic CS) cannot be found. Bilateral adrenalectomy is generally advisable in patients with bilateral ACTH-independent (macro- or micronodular) adrenal hyperplasia. Patients require lifelong glucocorticoid and mineralocorticoid replacement after bilateral adrenalectomy. Monitor for Nelson's syndrome (corticotroph tumor progression) with regular ACTH levels and pituitary MRI examinations in patients with CD who undergo bilateral adrenalectomy.

Minimize Glucocorticoid Exposure in Patients with Iatrogenic Cushing's Syndrome

In patients with iatrogenic CS, minimize the glucocorticoid doses as needed to treat the underlying illness. If possible, avoid ritonavir or cobicistat in patients on long-term glucocorticoids. For those patients on long-term steroids who no longer require pharmacologic doses, prescribe replacement doses (equivalent of prednisone 3–5 mg/day), with appropriate stress-dose coverage at the time of surgery or acute illness, until recovery of the hypothalamic-pituitary-adrenal (HPA) axis occurs. Although practice varies, clinicians will often monitor morning plasma cortisol (prior to steroid dose) or perform ACTH stimulation testing to document recovery of the HPA axis.

The Diagnosis and Management of Cushing's Syndrome in Pregnancy Are Challenging but Tumor-Directed Surgery Remains First-Line Therapy and Can Be Life-Saving

Making the diagnosis is critical as CS in pregnancy is associated with significant morbidity and mortality for the fetus and mother. Do not use the DST. Use the UFC with a higher cutoff of 2–3 × prepregnancy ULN, since cortisol secretion rates rise during healthy pregnancies above pregestational levels. The LNSC may be useful, but more data are needed on reference ranges. Adrenal causes are proportionately more common during pregnancy (~50% of CS), but ACTH may not be fully suppressed. Order an abdominal ultrasound as the initial imaging modality; unenhanced MRI of the adrenals or pituitary may be performed in consultation with radiology. Tumor-directed surgery, preferably during the second trimester, should be undertaken if a source is identified. No pharmacotherapy is approved for use in pregnancy; metyrapone has been used the most, but cabergoline may also be useful. Mifepristone is absolutely contraindicated as it is an abortifacient.

Suggested Reading

Elamin MB, Murad MH, Mullan R, Erickson D, Harris K, Nadeem S, et al. Accuracy of diagnostic tests for Cushing's syndrome: a systematic review and metaanalyses. J Clin Endocrinol Metabol. 2008;93(5):1553–62.

Lacroix A, Feelders RA, Stratakis CA, Nieman LK. Cushing's syndrome. Lancet (Lond, Engl). 2015;386(9996):913–27.

Nieman LK, Biller BMK, Findling JW, Murad MH, Newell-Price J, Savage MO, et al. Treatment of Cushing's syndrome: an endocrine society clinical practice guideline. J Clin Endocrinol Metabol. 2015;100(8):2807–31.

Nieman LK, Biller BMK, Findling JW, Newell-Price J, Savage MO, Stewart PM, et al. The diagnosis of Cushing's syndrome: an endocrine society clinical practice guideline. J Clin Endocrinol Metabol. 2008;93(5):1526–40.

Pivonello R, De Leo M, Cozzolino A, Colao A. The treatment of Cushing's disease. Endocr Rev. 2015;36(4):385–486.

Tritos N, Biller BMK. Medical therapy for Cushing's syndrome in the twenty-first century. Endocrinol Metab Clin N Am. 2018;47(2):427–40.

Adrenalectomy

19

Ole-Petter R. Hamnvik

Contents

Abbreviation

IV   Intravenous

O.-P. R. Hamnvik (✉)
Brigham and Women's Hospital, Department of Medicine, Division
of Endocrinology, Diabetes and Hypertension, Boston, MA, USA
e-mail: ohamnvik@bwh.harvard.edu

© Springer Nature Switzerland AG 2020   229
R. K. Garg et al. (eds.), *Handbook of Inpatient Endocrinology*,
https://doi.org/10.1007/978-3-030-38976-5_19

Preoperative Evaluation

Review Indications for Adrenalectomy and Consider Appropriateness of a Biopsy

Most adrenal masses should not be surgically removed. Indications for unilateral adrenalectomy include:

- Hormonally secreting adrenal adenomas (such as cortisol-producing or aldosterone-producing adenomas)

- Pheochromocytomas
- Adrenal masses that are suspicious for primary adrenocortical carcinoma, based on imaging characteristics such as irregular shape, size >4 cm, high unenhanced CT attenuation values (>20 Hounsfield units), irregular enhancement after contrast administration, etc.
- As part of a radical nephrectomy for renal cell carcinoma or other rarer tumors such as Wilms tumor or neuroblastomas

Bilateral adrenalectomy is usually only performed in the setting of ACTH-dependent Cushing syndrome where the source of the ACTH excess cannot be identified or controlled (such as in a widely metastatic ACTH-secreting malignancy).

Adrenalectomy is usually not performed for non-adrenal cancer with metastatic spread to the adrenal gland or for infections causing adrenal masses such as tuberculosis, fungi, etc. Therefore, a fine needle aspiration biopsy may be reasonable if there is concern for metastasis (such as in a patient with a known primary tumor) or infection (such as in a patient with systemic symptoms such as fevers, chills, weight loss, etc.). Biopsy should not be performed until pheochromocytoma has been ruled out biochemically. In addition, biopsy will not distinguish adrenocortical cancer from an adrenal adenoma (a full resection is required) and therefore is not indicated in suspected adreno-cortical cancer.

The indication for surgery, the surgeon's experience, and characteristics of the patient and the tumor will determine the surgical approach chosen by the surgeon. The standard approach for benign disease is laparoscopic transabdominal adrenalectomy or retroperitoneal endoscopic adrenalectomy. These approaches are used in the vast majority of adrenalectomies and are considered the standard of care for adrenalectomies for benign lesions, particularly in patients who are otherwise at high risk for postoperative complications. Open transabdominal adrenalectomy is a more invasive surgical approach that allows the best exposure and visualization of the operative field; it is usually the preferred approach in cases of suspected malignancy where a more extensive resection is needed. This includes cases of known adrenocortical carcinoma, suspected adrenocortical carcinoma (such as tumors >6 cm in size, tumors making multiple hormones, or tumors making adrenal androgens), and tumors with local invasion into surrounding structures. However, the open approach to adrenalectomy is associated with more pain and longer postoperative hospitalization than less invasive approaches, although this is a reasonable trade-off to allow more complete resection in cases of suspected malignancy.

Ensure Completeness of Preoperative Endocrine Evaluation

All patients with an adrenal mass should have an evaluation for hormonal hypersecretion by history, physical examination, and biochemical testing prior to surgery. If adrenalectomy is performed in a patient without an adrenal mass (such as in a radical nephrectomy), an endocrine evaluation is not required unless the patient has an incidental adrenal mass noted on preoperative imaging.

The history and physical examination should focus on symptoms and signs of Cushing syndrome, primary hyperaldosteronism (mainly by assessing blood pressure), androgen excess, and pheochromocytoma. All patients with an adrenal nodule should have a biochemical assessment for Cushing syndrome (1-mg dexamethasone suppression test or late-night salivary cortisol level) and pheochromocytoma (plasma or 24-h urine metanephrines). Patients with hypertension or hypokalemia should also be assessed for primary aldosteronism with an aldosterone-renin ratio. When adrenocortical carcinoma is suspected, andorgen levels should be measured: primarily DHEAS, but also consider testosterone and androstenedione. Males and post-menopausal females with features of estrogen excess should have estogen levels measured.

Assessing the endocrine function preoperatively is essential to avoid unexpected intraoperative or postoperative complications. Patients who have preoperative cortisol excess from a cortisol-secreting adrenal adenoma are at risk for adrenal insufficiency postoperatively due to atrophy of pituitary corticotrophs and of the contralateral adrenal gland; they are also at higher risk of venous thromboembolism, hyperglycemia, hypertension, peptic ulcer disease, and infection. Perioperative management of these patients is discussed in Chap. 18 "Cushing's Syndrome." Patients with primary aldosteronism may need preoperative blood pressure control and hypokalemia treatment (often with a mineralocorticoid receptor antagonist such as spironolactone) and are at risk for postoperative hypoaldosteronism with hyperkalemia and sodium wasting with hypotension, as discussed in Chap. 21 "Primary Aldosteronism." Patients with pheochromocytomas should receive preoperative blockade of alpha- and beta-Adrenergic receptors as well as volume expansion, as discussed in Chap. 20 "Pheochromocytoma and Paraganglioma," to prevent uncontrollable intraoperative blood pressure swings. A finding of hyperandrogenism raises the likelihood that the lesion is an adrenocortical cancer; benign adrenal adenomas almost never secrete androgens.

Postoperative Management

Assess for Hormonal Deficiencies

Postoperatively, adrenal insufficiency may be an expected occurrence, such as after bilateral adrenalectomy. These patients do not need any further hormonal assessment but should start hormone replacement as discussed below. In patients who have undergone unilateral adrenalectomy for a hormonally silent lesion, as assessed preoperatively, the likelihood of clinically apparent adrenal insufficiency is low, and routine glucocorticoid replacement is therefore not indicated. However, biochemical adrenal insufficiency on postoperative day 1 (defined by a morning cortisol below 94 nmol/L [3.4 µg/dL]) has been found in around 20% of patients and may represent suppression of the remaining adrenal from subclinical Cushing syndrome or an inadequate adrenocortical reserve in the remaining adrenal. While routine postoperative testing for adrenal insufficiency in these patients is not currently standard of care, close monitoring of the patient's clinical status (symptoms, blood pressure, electrolytes) should be performed, and there should be a low threshold to assess for adrenal insufficiency. Postoperative endocrine monitoring of patients with secretory adrenal masses is discussed in Chap. 18 "Cushing's Syndrome," Chap. 20 "Pheochromocytoma and Paraganglioma," and Chap. 21 "Primary Hyperaldosteronism."

Initiate Replacement Therapy

Patients who undergo bilateral adrenalectomy, as well as those patients whose indication for unilateral adrenalectomy is a cortisol-secreting adrenal adenoma or adenocarcinoma, will have adrenal insufficiency postoperatively. Therefore, routine administration of glucocorticoids is indicated.

For patients who have undergone bilateral adrenalectomy, an example of a postoperative hormone replacement strategy is the following:

- Hydrocortisone 50 mg IV every 8 h on the day of surgery and postoperative day 1, with the first dose being administered intraoperatively after the second adrenal gland has been removed.
- Then reduce the dose to 25 mg IV every 8 h on postoperative day 2.
- On postoperative day 3, if the patient is tolerating oral intake, switch to oral hydrocortisone, 40 mg at 7 am and 20 mg at 3 pm for 1 day and then to 20 mg at 7 am and 10 mg at 3 pm thereafter. When oral intake is tolerated, oral fludrocortisone 0.1 mg daily is also added.
- The dose can be weaned further after discharge based on patient symptoms, blood pressure readings and potassium levels.

In patients who have undergone adrenal surgery for overt or subclinical cortisol excess, some practitioners prefer to wait with initiation of glucocorticoids until postoperative day 1 after ensuring that blood cortisol levels have dropped, confirming surgical cure of the disease. In patients with overt Cushing syndrome, higher supraphysiologic glucocorticoid doses and a slower taper are often needed as the patient can otherwise be very symptomatic from the rapid decline in glucocorticoid levels. Patients who undergo unilateral adrenalectomy for any indication usually do not require mineralocorticoid replacement with fludrocortisone, although they should be monitored for hyperkalemia and hypotension which are signs of hypoaldosteronism.

Educate the Patient About Adrenal Insufficiency if Present

All patients diagnosed with adrenal insufficiency should be informed about their diagnosis and taught how to prevent adrenal crises prior to discharge. This is discussed in further detail in Chap. 17 "Suspected Adrenocortical Deficiency."

Organize Follow-Up After Discharge

Patients should have a follow-up appointment within 1–2 weeks with their surgeon for routine postoperative follow-up and to discuss the results of the histopathologic examination of the adrenal specimen. Patients who are diagnosed with adrenocortical cancer or patients who are discharged on adrenal hormone replacement should have follow-up with an endocrinologist within 2–4 weeks to discuss whether adjuvant mitotane is indicated and to titrate the hormone replacement dose, respectively. Patients should have a contact number in case symptoms of adrenal insufficiency develop.

Suggested Reading

Fassnacht M, Arlt W, Bancos I, Dralle H, Newell-Price J, Sahdev A, et al. Management of adrenal incidentalomas: European Society of Endocrinology Clinical Practice Guideline in collaboration with the European Network for the Study of Adrenal Tumors. Eur J Endocrinol. 2016;175(2):G1–G34.

Mitchell J, Barbosa G, Tsinberg M, Milas M, Siperstein A, Berber E. Unrecognized adrenal insufficiency in patients undergoing laparoscopic adrenalectomy. Surg Endosc. 2009;23:248–54.

Zeiger MA, Thompson GB, Duh QY, Hamrahian AH, Angelos P, Elaraj D, et al. The American Association of Clinical Endocrinologists and American Association of Endocrine Surgeons medical guidelines for the management of adrenal incidentalomas. Endocr Pract. 2009;15(Suppl 1):1–20.

Pheochromocytoma and Paraganglioma

20

Alejandro Raul Ayala
and Mark Anthony Jara

Contents

A. R. Ayala (✉)
University of Miami, Miller School of Medicine, Department
of Endocrinology and Metabolism, Miami, FL, USA
e-mail: aayala2@miami.edu

M. A. Jara
University of Miami, Miller School of Medicine, Division
of Endocrinology and Metabolism, Miami, FL, USA
e-mail: maj158@miami.edu

© Springer Nature Switzerland AG 2020
R. K. Garg et al. (eds.), *Handbook of Inpatient Endocrinology*,
https://doi.org/10.1007/978-3-030-38976-5_20

Before the Admission

Because pheochromocytoma and catecholamine-secreting paragangliomas (PPGLs) might have similar clinical presentations and are treated with similar approaches, many clinicians use the term "pheochromocytoma" to refer to both. The most common inpatient consultation often involves perioperative management of a patient previously diagnosed with a pheochromocytoma. However, catecholamine secreting tumors can also be diagnosed during a hospitalization for unrelated conditions or in the context of a hypertensive crisis. The clinical presentation of patients with PPGLs varies widely from no symptoms or minor discrete symptoms to catastrophic life-threatening clinical conditions. In general, 50% of these patients are asymptomatic at presentation. This subgroup is much larger in those patients with incidentally discovered adrenal masses or those tested during family screenings. When symptomatic, patients may present with the following:

- Pounding headache, approximately 90% of symptomatic patients.
- Profuse sweating in 60–70%.
- Palpitations that occurs in spells that last from several minutes to 1 h with complete remission of the symptoms between spells. The spells could occur either spontaneously or being provoked by a variety of physical or chemical triggers, such as general anesthesia, micturition, and medications (e.g., β-adrenergic inhibitors, tricyclic antidepressants, glucocorticoids).
- Panic attack like symptoms.

Approximately 50% of patients have paroxysmal hypertension, often severe, while the remaining either have primary hypertension or are normotensive (5–15%). Other symptoms include tremors, pallor, dyspnea, weakness mostly generalized, and panic attack-type symptoms. On rare occasion, catecholamine excess can result in decompensated heart failure and/or cardiogenic shock with features of stress-induced (Takotsubo) cardiomyopathy.

Preoperative Blood Pressure Control

The main goal of preoperative management of a pheochromocytoma patient is to normalize blood pressure, heart rate, and function of other organs; restore volume depletion; and prevent a patient from surgery-induced catecholamine storm and its potentially devastating consequences.

All patients with a biochemically positive pheochromocytoma should receive appropriate preoperative medical management to block the effects of released catecholamines. Medical treatment should be started ideally 14 days preoperatively allowing for blood pressure and pulse normalization. Based on retrospective studies and institutional experience, target goals include a blood pressure of less than 130/80 mm Hg while seated and greater than 90 mm Hg systolic while standing and a heart rate target of 60–70 bpm seated and 70–80 bpm standing.

The α-adrenergic receptor blockers are the first-choice agents having significant impact on surgical outcome as patients without α-adrenoceptor blockade experience significant perioperative complications when compared with those on treatment. Phenoxybenzamine (a noncompetitive, α-adrenoceptor blocker) is most commonly used for preoperative blockade. The initial dose of phenoxybenzamine is usually 10 mg twice a day followed by 10–20 mg increments every 2–3 days until the clinical manifestations are controlled or further increases are limited by side effects. Generally, a total daily dose of 1 mg/kg is sufficient. Additionally, the prolonged action of phenoxybenzamine can contribute to hypotension in the first 24 h after tumor removal. Another option is to administer phenoxybenzamine by infusion (0.5 mg/kg·d) for 5 h a day, 3 days before the surgical intervention in those patients that are hospitalized. Prazosin, terazosin, and doxazosin are specific competitive alpha 1-postsynaptic blocking α-adrenoceptor blocking agents of shorter half-life that can also be used safely. Prazosin is administered in doses of 2–5 mg two or three times a day, terazosin in doses of 2–5 mg per day, and doxazosin in doses of 2–8 mg per day. These three medications could potentially induce severe postural hypotension immediately after the first dose; thus, they should be given just as the patient is ready to go to bed. Thereafter, the dosage can be increased as needed; titration can be achieved more quickly with much less side effects compared with phenoxybenzamine.

Beta-adrenoceptor blocking agents are needed when catecholamine-related or α-blocker-induced tachyarrhythmia occurs but should never be used before an adequate α-blockade has been established as unopposed alpha-receptor stimulation will cause increased vasoconstriction and might lead to hypertensive crisis.

Calcium channel blockers may also be used preoperatively. The combination of extended-release verapamil (180–360 mg/ daily), sustained release nicardipine beginning with 30 mg twice daily, amlodipine beginning with 2.5-5 mg daily or extended release nifedipine beginning with 30 mg daily and specific competitive alpha 1-postsynaptic α-adrenoceptor blocking agents (i.e., doxazosin) may be particularly useful although there is little data to compare the efficacy of one treatment regimen over another. Calcium channel blockers do not cause hypotension or orthostatic hypotension during normotensive period and may also be used as the primary preoperative treatment of choice in normotensive patients with pheochromocytoma. These agents may also prevent catecholamine-associated coronary spasm; therefore, they may be useful when pheochromocytoma is associated with catecholamine-induced coronary vasospasm.

Hydration

Adequate oral hydration should be encouraged prior to admission. Catecholamines cause intense vasoconstriction through the alpha-1 receptors, and initiation of α-blockade can lead to severe orthostatic hypotension. A patient may need 2–3 L of fluid orally or intravenously with 5–10 g of salt to increase the intravascular volume, reverse catecholamine-induced blood volume contraction preoperatively, and prevent severe hypotension after tumor removal. Serial hematocrit measurements give a guide to the effectiveness of volume expansion. Usually, a 5–10% fall in hematocrit is seen in well-prepared patients.

During Admission

Inpatient Diagnosis and Treatment

The diagnosis of a pheochromocytoma in hospitalized patients can be challenging, mainly due to confounders that can result in non-tumoral catecholamine elevation. Coexisting conditions (heart failure, renal failure, and hypoglycemia) increase sympathetic activity and may result in a false-positive test. Interfering medications and psychiatric conditions should also be taken into account. Confirmatory biochemical testing should generally precede imaging procedures because only solid evidence of excess production of catecholamines can justify performing expensive imaging procedures. However, a highly suspicious lesion (i.e., markedly hyperintense vascular tumor on T2 MRI images with no signal loss on out-of-phase imaging) should prompt immediate and incisive investigation. Imaging characteristics are particularly important during the evaluation of an incidentally discovered adrenal tumor (adrenal incidentaloma), since the tumor may be in the so called pre-biochemical phase (normal catecholamines/metanephrines).

Initial biochemical testing for PPGLs should include measurements of plasma-free metanephrines or urinary fractionated metanephrines by either mass spectrometry, liquid chromatography with electrochemical, or fluorometric detection (LC-ECD), as they have shown superior sensitivity and accuracy compared to VMA and urine catecholamines. For measurement of plasma metanephrines, it is recommended to test the patient in the supine position and use of reference intervals established in the same position. An elevation of two to four times above the normal reference values often confirms the diagnosis with few exceptions.

Confounders: Diagnostic Accuracy of Metanephrines

Plasma (free and total) metanephrines have similar sensitivities of 96% and 95% to urinary fractionated metanephrines. Both tests are equally recommended and combination of tests is not necessary. To avoid false positives, acetaminophen should be avoided for 5 days before blood sampling (HPLC assay). Caffeine intake and cigarette smoking should be discontinued for at least 24 h before a blood sample is obtained. The blood sample should be drawn in lavender or green-top tube, transferred on ice, and then stored at −80 °C until analyzed. The highest diagnostic sensitivity for plasma-free metanephrines is reached if the collection is performed in the supine position after an overnight fast and while the patient is recumbent in a quiet room for at least 20–30 min (Table 20.1).

Table 20.1 Drugs that can affect the levels of plasma and urinary catecholamines or metanephrines and affect test accuracy

Medications	Effect
Tricyclic antidepressants amitriptyline, imipramine, and nortriptyline	Increase plasma and urinary NA, NMA, and VMA
SSRI	Increased NMA
Blockers atenolol, propranolol	Increase plasma MA
Caffeine, nicotine	Increase plasma and urinary A and NA
Calcium channel antagonists	Increase plasma A and NA
Amphetamine, ephedrine	Increase plasma and urinary A and NA
SNRI (venlafaxine)	Increase NMA

Adapted from Davison AS. Biochemical Investigations in Laboratory Medicine. Physiological effects of medications on Plasma/Urine metanephrines. Newcastle upon Tyne NHS Foundation Trust. http://www.pathology.leedsth.nhs.uk/dnn_bilm/Misc/Effectofdrugsonmetanephrines.aspx. (See Suggested Readings)

NA noradrenaline, *A* adrenaline, *NMA* normetadrenaline, *MA* metadrenaline, *VMA* vanillylmandelic acid

Localization of Pheochromocytomas/PPGLs

Localization of PPGLs is only done when there is biochemical diagnosis confirmation. CT or MRI may be used as the usual initial imaging modalities for localization of PPGLs. These studies have high sensitivity but less than optimal specificity. These should be combined with functional imaging studies (nuclear medicine) to rule out extra-adrenal pheochromocytoma or metastatic disease. Gallium-68 PET/C is a promising agent that may offer further advantage in the localization of paragangliomas (Fig. 20.1).

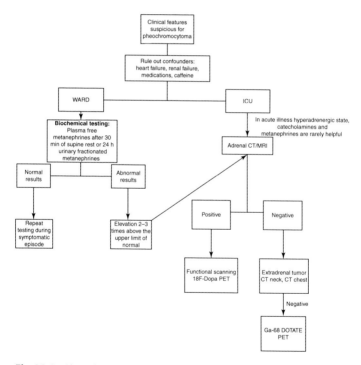

Fig. 20.1 *Algorithm 1* Biochemical and imaging diagnosis of catecholamine-producing tumors

Opportunities to Explore Syndromic Pheochromocytoma: Hints of Genotype

Pheochromocytoma/PPGLs may be inherited and may have distinct characteristic setting them apart from sporadic pheochromocytoma. Patients with syndromic lesions and/or positive family history should be tested for appertaining genes.

Considerations should be made in patient presenting with:

- PPGL at young age, usually before 40 years old
- Positive family history
- Multifocal PPGLs
- Bilateral adrenal tumors

Pheochromocytomas are associated with the following familial syndromes: multiple endocrine neoplasia type 2 (MEN 2), von Hippel-Lindau disease (VHL), von Recklinghausen's neurofibromatosis type 1 (NF 1), and familial paragangliomas (PGLs).

Hospitalization represents a unique opportunity to identify such associated syndromic inherited conditions. Furthermore, the presence of family members providing support to the hospitalized patient represents an opportunity to further explore familial forms and to evaluate family members following appropriate consent.

Anesthesia in the Patient with Pheochromocytoma

Pheochromocytoma represents an important challenge for the anesthesiologist. By some estimates, 25–50% of hospital deaths of patients with unmanaged or unknown pheochromocytoma occur during induction of anesthesia or during operative procedures for other conditions, mostly related to lethal hypertensive crises, malignant arrhythmias, and multiorgan failure. Most patients with pheochromocytoma will require surgical intervention, and labile blood pressures, arrhythmias, and tachycardia during and after surgery are not uncommon. Risks are much higher for patients with unrecognized pheochromocytoma who undergo anesthesia for unrelated surgery. Multidisciplinary preoperative evaluation and medical management before surgery are important.

Once the diagnosis is confirmed, medical management for surgery preparation is recommended as resecting a pheochromocytoma is a high-risk surgical procedure.

Preoperative cardiac evaluation should include an electrocardiogram (ECG) to evaluate for possible ischemic changes and rhythm disturbances as damage to the cardiovascular system is the most likely to impact on outcomes in patient requiring anesthesia.

A number of medications commonly used in anesthesia should be avoided or used cautiously in patients with pheochromocytoma. Metoclopramide is associated with hypertensive crisis and adrenergic myocarditis with cardiogenic shock in patients with pheochromocytoma. Phenothiazine derivatives, including droperidol, haloperidol, and chlorpromazine, can result in hypotension in patients with pheochromocytoma. Glucagon has been shown to release catecholamines from the tumor and also linked with hypertensive crisis (Fig. 20.2).

Early Postoperative

The postoperative management usually requires an intensive care unit admission as once the tumor is removed the withdrawal of catecholamine effect will result in hypotension. The incidence of hypotension is variably described as 20–70% in various reports and may somewhat be dependent on the use of nature of preoperative alpha-antagonist and intraoperative hypotensive agents. Fluid replacement and vasopressor infusion might be necessary in some patients. After tumor removal, sudden catecholamine withdrawal can lead to severe hypoglycemia, and blood sugar monitoring, at least for the initial 12–24 h of the postoperative period, is recommended.

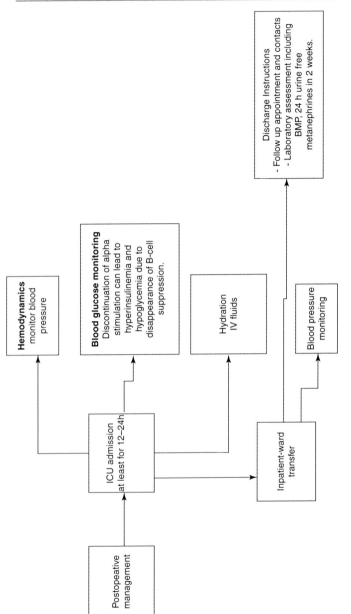

Fig. 20.2 *Algorithm 2* Postoperative management of pheochromocytoma

Special Circumstances

The Pregnant Patient

Pheochromocytoma has a reported incidence of <0.2 per 10,000 pregnancies. Although a rare disorder, untreated, it carries a risk of mortality for both mother and fetus. Pheochromocytomas have the ability to produce signs and symptoms that mimic other forms of hypertension, including the new-onset hypertensive syndromes in pregnancy, gestational hypertension, and preeclampsia. It may become overt during pregnancy because of increases in intra-abdominal pressure, fetal movements, uterine contractions, the process of delivery, an abdominal surgical intervention, and even general anesthesia.

The diagnosis is based on the results of 24-h urinary fractionated metanephrines and/or plasma fractionated metanephrines. MRI without gadolinium is the preferred imaging modality for localization as it locates adrenal and extra-adrenal masses and requires no radiation.

The management has primary goal to prevent hypertensive crisis. Medical treatment with α-blockers must be started as soon as the diagnosis is confirmed and should be given for 10–14 days. The drug of choice is phenoxybenzamine (pregnancy class C), followed by a β-blocker if necessary. Phenoxybenzamine crosses the placenta and may cause perinatal depression in the mother and transient hypotension in the neonate; however, it has been described as generally safe for the fetus. Methyldopa is not recommended, because it may worsen the symptoms of pheochromocytoma. Cesarean section is the preferred mode of delivery since it appears to carry less risk of maternal death than vaginal delivery. The definitive treatment is surgery, and tumor resection can be completed either before 24 weeks, as second trimester is the safest period to do surgery during pregnancy, or a few weeks later after uterine involution.

The ICU Patient

Because critical illness results in a hyperadrenergic state, measurements of catecholamines and metanephrines are rarely helpful in the ICU setting. Furthermore, vasoactive amines and antiarrhythmics may also interfere with diagnostic testing. Therefore, a CT of the abdomen with emphasis on the adrenal gland may be the most convenient test in this situation, as most pheochromocytomas are large (4–5 cm) and have distinct imaging characteristics.

Renal Failure

Measurements of urinary catecholamines and metabolites are less reliable if the patient has advanced kidney disease. In addition, serum chromogranin A levels have poor specificity in these patients. There is very limited literature in this regard. However, one study by Eisenhofer G et al. found that in renal failure, there are up to twofold higher plasma concentrations of catecholamines and free metanephrines.

Suggested Reading

Amar L, Bertherat J, Baudin E, Ajzenberg C, Bressac-de Paillerets B, Chabre O, et al. Genetic testing in pheochromocytoma or functional paraganglioma. J Clin Oncol. 2005;23(34):8812–8.

Barrett C, van Uum SH, Lenders JW. Risk of catecholaminergic crisis following glucocorticoid administration in patients with an adrenal mass: a literature review. Clin Endocrinol (Oxf). 2015;83(5):622–8.

Davison AS. Biochemical investigations in laboratory medicine. Physiological effects of medications on plasma/urine metanephrines. Newcastle upon Tyne NHS Foundation Trust. http://www.pathology.leedsth.nhs.uk/dnn_bilm/Misc/Effectofdrugsonmetanephrines.aspx.

Eisenhofer G, Peitzsch M. Laboratory evaluation of pheochromocytoma and paraganglioma. Clin Chem. 2014;60(12):1486–99.

Eisenhofer G, Rivers G, Rosas AL, Quezado Z, Manger WM, Pacak K. Adverse drug reactions in patients with pheochromocytoma: incidence, prevention and management. Drug Saf. 2007;30(11):1031–62.

Lenders JW, Duh QY, Eisenhofer G, Gimenez-Roqueplo AP, Grebe SK, Murad MH, et al. Pheochromocytoma and paraganglioma: an endocrine society clinical practice guideline. Endocrine Society. J Clin Endocrinol Metabol. 2014;99(6):1915–42.

Manger WM, Gifford RW. Pheochromocytoma. J Clin Hypertens (Greenwich). 2002;4(1):62–72.

Pacak K. Preoperative management of the pheochromocytoma patient. J Clin Endocrinol Metabol. 2007;92(11):4069–79.

Pacak K, Eisenhofer G, Ahlman H, Bornstein SR, Gimenez-Roqueplo AP, Grossman AB, et al. International Symposium on Pheochromocytoma. 2005 Pheochromocytoma: recommendations for clinical practice from the First International Symposium. Nat Clin Pract Endocrinol Metab. 2007;3(2):92–102.

Primary Aldosteronism

21

Alejandro Raul Ayala
and Mark Anthony Jara

Contents

A. R. Ayala (✉)
University of Miami, Miller School of Medicine, Department of Endocrinology and Metabolism, Miami, FL, USA
e-mail: aayala2@miami.edu

M. A. Jara
University of Miami, Miller School of Medicine, Division of Endocrinology and Metabolism, Miami, FL, USA
e-mail: maj158@med.miami.edu

© Springer Nature Switzerland AG 2020
R. K. Garg et al. (eds.), *Handbook of Inpatient Endocrinology*,
https://doi.org/10.1007/978-3-030-38976-5_21

Diagnostic Considerations

Primary aldosteronism (PA) is the most common cause of endocrine hypertension. Patients with PA have higher cardiovascular morbidity and mortality compared with age- and sex-matched patients with essential hypertension and the same degree of blood pressure elevation.

Case detection screening should be considered in patients with:

- Spontaneous hypokalemia, including patients treated with low-dose thiazide diuretics. However, there are patients with primary mineralocorticoid excess who are normokalemic and rarely some who are hypokalemic but normotensive. Only 9–37% of patients with primary aldosteronism are hypokalemic.
- Severe or resistant hypertension to three conventional antihypertensive drugs (including a diuretic) or controlled BP (<140/90 mm Hg) requiring four or more antihypertensive drugs.
- Patients with hypertension and adrenal incidentaloma.
- Hypertension and a family history of early-onset hypertension or cerebrovascular accident at a young age (<40 years).
- Hypertensive first-degree relatives of patients with PA.

Inpatient Testing for Hyperaldosteronism

The recommended case detection-screening test is the plasma aldosterone activity (PAC)/plasma renin activity (PRA).

An elevated plasma aldosterone activity (PAC)/plasma renin activity (PRA) ratio and an increased PAC are required for the diagnosis of primary aldosteronism.

- PAC is inappropriately high for the PRA, usually >15 ng/dL.
- PAC/PRA ratio greater than 20.

Collecting blood midmorning from seated patients following 2–4-h upright posture improves sensitivity.

In the setting of spontaneous hypokalemia, plasma renin below detection levels plus plasma aldosterone concentration (PAC) >20 ng/dL, further confirmatory testing might not be needed.

Confirmatory Testing Usually, elevated PAC/PRA ratio alone does not establish the diagnosis of primary aldosteronism, and the results have to be confirmed by demonstrating inappropriate aldosterone secretion, except in situations as spontaneous hypokalemia, undetectable PRA or PRC, and a PAC >20 ng/dL. Otherwise, aldosterone suppression testing is needed with one of several tests (table of confirmatory test).

The patient that presents with hypertensive crisis despite the use of multiple antihypertensives should be screened for primary hyperaldosteronism.

Factors Affecting Aldosterone/Renin Ratio

False Negatives Genrally limited to the mineralocorticoid receptor antagonists, spironolactone and eplerenone. While dietary salt restriction, concomitant malignant or renovascular hypertension, pregnancy, and treatment with diuretics (including spironolactone), dihydropyridine calcium blockers, angiotensin-converting enzyme inhibitors, and angiotensin receptor antagonists can stimulate renin, they generally do not have a sufficiently potent effect to interfere with diagnosing PA.

False Positives Beta-blockers, alpha-methyldopa, clonidine, and nonsteroidal anti-inflammatory drugs suppress renin, raising the ARR with potential for false positives. False positives can also occur in patient with advanced age and renal disease.

In general, medications other than the minetarlocorticoid antagonists do not need to be discontinued before ARR measurement. However, when the diagnosis is not clear, the interfering medications should be discontinued at least 2 weeks before ARR measurement; diuretics should be discontinued ideally 6 weeks before the test, although this is inconvenient, potentially harmful and rarely feasible. Some patients will require substitution of the interfering medication during the washout period until the test is completed. Doxazosin and fosinopril can be used in hypertensive patients who need to undergo aldosterone and PRA measurement for the diagnosis of primary aldosteronism; amlodipine yields a small percentage of false-negative diagnoses, and beta-blockers may only have limited influence on the diagnosis of primary aldosteronism as they lower PRA and PRC measurements and raise the PAC/PRA ratio, an effect that in most settings is not clinically significant. Other potassium-sparing diuretics, such as amiloride and triamterene, usually do not interfere with testing unless the patient is treated with high doses.

Special Considerations: Cortisol Co-secretion

There is an increasing awareness of cortisol co-secretion in the context of primary hyperaldosteronism resulting from adrenal tumors. Overt or subtle glucocorticoid hypersecretion may potentially interfere with diagnostic studies or result in secondary/tertiary adrenal insufficiency after surgical removal of the tumor because of contralateral gland suppression. Patients with adrenal tumors, including those with confirmed hyperaldosteronism, should also be evaluated for hypercortisolism with a 1 mg dexamethasone suppression test.

Disease Subtyping

Once the diagnosis of primary hyperaldosteronism has been confirmed, unilateral adenoma or rarely carcinoma must be distinguished from bilateral disease. Disease subtyping is established using adrenal computed tomography (CT) and adrenal vein sampling (AVS) (algorithm). Adrenal vein sampling is used to distinguish between unilateral adenoma and bilateral hyperplasia, and it is recommended to confirm unilateral secretion for patients who would likely pursue surgical management.

Treatment

The curative treatment is surgical: unilateral laparoscopic adrenalectomy for patients with documented unilateral PA or unilateral adrenal hyperplasia.

Medical treatment is preferred in patients who are unable or unwilling to undergo surgery or who have bilateral adrenal disease. Mineralocorticoid receptor antagonists are the medical treatment of choice. Spironolactone is the primary agent at doses ranging from 25 to 400 mg/d, with eplerenone as an alternative. Antiandrogen side effects such as gynecomastia and diminished libido in men and menstrual disorders in women can result from spironolactone due to cross-antagonism of the sex steroid receptor. Eplerenone is more specific for the aldosterone receptor and therefore causes less undesired side effects but is less potent than spironolactone. In a study comparing these two therapies, spironolactone at doses ranging from 75 to 225 mg/d was more efficacious than eplerenone at doses between 100 and 300 mg/d for hypertension control. Biochemical cure following adrenalectomy as well as hemodynamic improvement is seen in over 90% of patients. Hypokalemia typically resolves immediately after surgery, and blood pressure reduction may take months, prompting a reduction in quantity of antihypertensive medications in most patients.

Early Postoperative Period

We suggest the measurement of aldosterone and PRA on the first and second postoperative day. A significant decrease in serum aldosterone levels is detected a few hours after adrenal clipping is performed during adrenalectomy, although plasma renin activity may take weeks to normalize.

In general, when the unilateral adrenalectomy is successful, aldosterone levels achieve a nadir within 24–48 h after the intervention, suggesting cure. After surgery, mineralocorticoid receptor antagonists should be withdrawn in the first postoperative day to avoid hyperkalemia. Antihypertensives should be administered base on the patient's postoperative blood pressure readings. One should expect a significant reduction in the number of antihypertensives and dosing in most cases. On occasion, normotension is observed in the early postoperative period, particularly in younger patients with less severe preoperative hypertension, although blood pressure normalization may take up to a year to occur. Unless the patient is persistently hypokalemic, postoperative hydration should include normal saline without potassium with careful monitoring of renal function, as a decrease in GFR is often seen following resolution of hyperaldosteronism, a condition that results in glomerular hyperfiltration. Preoperative renal damage as revealed by elevated serum creatinine and microalbuminuria are significant predictors of postoperative hyperkalemia (hypoaldosteronism).

Hence, the combination of worsening renal function and post-surgical hypoaldosteronism that occurs in cured patients treated with unilateral adrenalectomy may result in severe hyperkalemia, requiring close attention not only in the early postoperative period but also following discharge. Because the hypoaldosteronism may be prolonged, we recommend at least weekly electrolyte and renal function testing during postsurgical month, as a minimum.

Special Considerations

Primary Hyperaldosteronisms and Pregnancy

Primary aldosteronism is uncommon in pregnancy, with only few cases reported in the literature, most of them due to aldosterone-producing adenomas. Primary aldosteronism can lead to intrauterine growth retardation, preterm delivery, intrauterine fetal demise, and placental abruption.

The evaluation in the pregnant woman is the same as for non-pregnant patients. For case confirmation, however, the captopril stimulation test is contraindicated in pregnancy, but measurement of sodium and aldosterone in a 24-h urine collection is an option. Subtype testing with abdominal magnetic resonance imaging (MRI) without gadolinium is the test of choice. Computed tomography (CT) and adrenal venous sampling are contraindicated in pregnancy.

Hypertension may improve or worsen in pregnancy due to the agonist/antagonist function of progesterone on the mineralocorticoid receptor.

The treatment depends on the case presentation including medical or surgical options:

- Unilateral laparoscopic adrenalectomy during the second trimester in clear cases of tumors of >1 cm.

- Spironolactone crosses the placenta and is a US Food and Drug Administration (FDA) pregnancy category C (Not proven safe in pregnancy), and eplerenone is an FDA pregnancy category B (There are no adequate and well-controlled studies in pregnant women. Should be used during pregnancy only if the potential benefit justifies the potential risk to the fetus). Therefore, standard antihypertensive drugs approved for use during pregnancy should be used.
- Hypokalemia can be managed with oral potassium supplements.

The Patient with Chronic Kidney Disease

The diagnosis of primary hyperaldosteronism could be challenging in patient with chronic kidney disease (CKD) as this may disturb the renin-angiotensin-aldosterone system. The diagnosis of primary PA in the CKD population has not been established as plasma aldosterone concentration, PRA, and ARR can vary significantly in CKD. As CKD progresses, PAC increases, and the more advanced the CKD, the lesser the effect on PRA, giving rise to a higher ARR. Also in a study, primary aldosteronism patients accompanying chronic kidney disease had high serum aldosterone and ARR levels, low PRA, and no clear association of hypokalemia.

Familial Hyperaldosteronism: Contact with the Family Members

Familial hyperaldosteronism is a group of inherited conditions inhered in an autosomal dominant pattern. Three familial forms of PA have been described:

- FH type I or glucocorticoid-remediable aldosteronism, usually associated with bilateral adrenal hyperplasia.
- FH type II is not dexamethasone suppressible.
- FH type III is caused by germ line mutations in the potassium channel subunit KCNJ5, mostly suspected in patient with massive adrenal hyperplasia and children.

The patient and their family should receive appropriate information as well as appropriate counseling for biochemical screening of family members; continuously updated databases of human genes and genetic disorders and traits like OMIM or MalaCards are excellent free educational resources (Fig. 21.1).

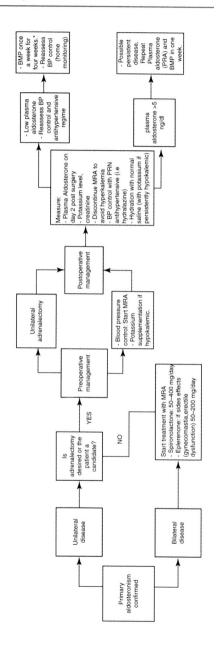

Fig. 21.1 *Algorithm:* inpatient management of primary hyperaldosteronism

* May require prolonged monitoring for persistent contralateral adrenocorticol supression (hypoaldosteronism)

MRA: Mineralocorticoid receptor antagonist   BP: Blood pressure   PRA: Plasma renin activity

Suggested Reading

Funder JW, Carey RM, Fardella C, Gomez-Sanchez CE, Mantero F, Stowasser M, Endocrine Society, et al. Case detection, diagnosis, and treatment of patients with primary aldosteronism: an Endocrine Society clinical practice guideline. J Clin Endocrinol Metabol. 2008;93(9):3266–81. https://doi.org/10.1210/jc.2008-0104.

Funder JW, Carey RM, Mantero F, Murad MH, Reincke M, Shibata H, et al. The management of primary aldosteronism: case detection, diagnosis, and treatment: an endocrine society clinical practice guideline. J Clin Endocrinol Metabol. 2016;101(5):1889–916. https://doi.org/10.1210/jc.2015-4061.

Keuer B, Ayala AR, Pinto P. The role of intra- and postoperative serum aldosterone levels following adrenalectomy for primary aldosteronism. 64th Annual Meeting of the American Urologic Association (Mid-Atlantic Section), Washington, DC, October 12–15 2006.

Mulatero P, Rabbia F, Milan A, Paglieri C, Morello F, Chiandussi L, Veglio F. Drug effects on aldosterone/plasma renin activity ratio in primary aldosteronism. Hypertension. 2002;40(6):897–902.

Parthasarathy HK, Ménard J, White WB, Young WF Jr, Williams GH, Williams B, et al. A double-blind, randomized study comparing the antihypertensive effect of eplerenone and spironolactone in patients with hypertension and evidence of primary aldosteronism. J Hypertens. 2011;29(5):980–90. https://doi.org/10.1097/HJH.0b013e3283455ca5.

Rossi GP, Auchus RJ, Brown M, Lenders JW, Naruse M, Plouin PF, et al. An expert consensus statement on use of adrenal vein sampling for the subtyping of primary aldosteronism. Hypertension. 2014;63(1):151–60. https://doi.org/10.1161/HYPERTENSIONAHA.113.02097.

Savard S, Amar L, Plouin PF, Steichen O. Cardiovascular complications associated with primary aldosteronism. A controlled cross-sectional study. Hypertension. 2013;62(2):331–6. https://doi.org/10.1161/HYPERTENSIONAHA.113.01060.

Stowasser M, Ahmed AH, Pimenta E, Taylor PJ, Gordon RD. Factors affecting the aldosterone/renin ratio. Horm Metab Res. 2012;44(3):170–6. https://doi.org/10.1055/s-0031-1295460.

Young WF. Primary aldosteronism: renaissance of a syndrome. Clin Endocrinol (Oxf). 2007;66(5):607–18.

Treatment of Hyperglycemia in a Hospitalized Patient Without Hyperglycemic Emergency

22

Rajesh K. Garg

Contents

R. K. Garg (✉)
Division of Endocrinology, Diabetes and Metabolism, University
of Miami Miller School of Medicine, Coral Gables, FL, USA
e-mail: rgarg@miami.edu

© Springer Nature Switzerland AG 2020
R. K. Garg et al. (eds.), *Handbook of Inpatient Endocrinology*,
https://doi.org/10.1007/978-3-030-38976-5_22

Obtain Hba1c Unless Available Within Last 3 Months

All hyperglycemic patients should get an HbA1c at the time of admission. HbA1c helps in diagnosing new-onset diabetes or assessing the preadmission diabetes control. It also helps in advising antidiabetic treatment at the time of discharge.

Assess Preadmission Diabetes Status and Antidiabetic Treatment

If possible, a detailed history including the duration of diabetes, type of diabetes, presence of complications of diabetes, and preadmission diabetes treatment, especially the use of insulin, should be obtained. A focused physical examination assessing body weight, presence of neuropathy, and peripheral vascular disease should be conducted.

Assess Current Nutritional Status

Many hospitalized patients are rendered nothing per-oral (NPO) at the time of admission due to an impending surgery or a diagnostic procedure or simply due to inability to eat. Make a note of the reason for NPO status and expected duration for this order.

Assess whether the patient will be able to swallow after lifting the NPO status and what type of foods are likely to be swallowed. Any special restrictions or additional requirements for food should be noted. Patients requiring special supplements in-between regular meals may require a modified insulin regimen. If a patient is getting enteral tube feed, note the content, rate, and times of tube feed. Similar data need to be collected for parenteral nutrition.

Assess Other Medications That May Affect Glycemic Status

Most hospitalized are likely to be receiving one or more medications that can potentially affect BG levels. Most important medications are agents like norepinephrine, dopamine, and glucocorticoids. If possible, medications for intravenous (IV) infusion should be prepared in glucose-free solutions rather than in dextrose water.

Point of Care (POC) Blood Glucose (BG) Monitoring

BG monitoring is often obtained using POC BG monitoring devices and is adequate for glycemic management in hospitalized patients. However, in the intensive care unit (ICU) setting, arterial blood glucose monitoring may be available if blood oxygen is being monitored at the same time. In a patient eating regular meals, BG monitoring should be ordered before meals and bedtime. In all other situations, blood glucose should be monitored at least every 6 h. More frequent monitoring may be appropriate in critically ill patients or in a rapidly changing clinical situation. POC monitoring devices are less accurate at low BG levels. Therefore, any BG value less than 70 mg/dl should be confirmed by sending a sample for plasma glucose to the central laboratory.

Insulin Infusion in Critically Ill Patients, Intraoperatively or During Labor/Delivery

Critically Ill Patients in Intensive Care Units

Most critically ill patients are NPO and have a rapidly changing clinical condition. The same may apply to some patients intraoperatively. Therefore, insulin infusion is the preferred treatment for these patients. All hospitals with an ICU should have an approved insulin infusion protocol that the entire ICU staff are familiar with. It is always better to order continuous insulin infusion using hospital approved protocol. Blood glucose should be monitored every 1–4 h and insulin infusion rate adjusted using an algorithm that takes into account the current insulin infusion rate, current BG levels, and the rate of rise or fall of BG level. Blood glucose targets may vary from one hospital to another but are usually in a range of 100–180 mg/dL. As the clinical condition improves, patients should be transitioned from insulin infusion to basal bolus insulin therapy. In most hospitals, general floors are not equipped to administer insulin infusion. Therefore, it is important to switch to basal-bolus insulin before the patient leaves the ICU.

Labor and Delivery

Hyperglycemia during labor and delivery increases the risk of hypoglycemia in the newborn because of beta cell stimulation by glucose diffusing from the placenta. Therefore, tight glycemic control with BG target 70–110 mg/dL is recommended during labor and delivery. Most women with pregestational type 1 diabetes require insulin and glucose infusion to maintain glycemic control. Women with type 2 diabetes and those with gestational diabetes may or may not require insulin infusion, but they need to be monitored hourly.

Order Correctional Insulin

Correctional insulin therapy, also called sliding scale insulin therapy, is ordered for almost all hospitalized patients with hyperglycemia who are not on an insulin infusion protocol. There has been much criticism of using correctional insulin alone in a patient with diabetes. It leads to highly fluctuating blood glucose levels with high risk of both hypoglycemia and hyperglycemia. Moreover, in a patient with type 1 diabetes or insulin-requiring type 2 diabetes, using sliding scale insulin alone can be dangerous because of the risk of diabetic ketoacidosis or hyperosmolar state. Therefore, correctional insulin therapy alone should be avoided, and it should be ordered along with basal or basal-bolus insulin therapy. However, in a non-insulin-dependent patient with mildly high BG levels after admission, it may be appropriate to order correctional insulin alone for 1–2 days while assessing the need for basal and nutritional insulin. Correctional insulin doses should be administered after each POC BG testing and, if possible, combined with nutritional insulin doses. Thus, insulin formulation used for correctional insulin should be the same as used for nutritional insulin. Correctional insulin doses should be administered in proportion to the total daily insulin doses: a lower scale for patients with total daily dose of insulin <40 units, medium scale for patients with total daily dose of insulin 41–80 units, and higher scale for those with total daily dose of insulin >80 units/day. Avoid using correctional insulin more frequently than every 4 h to prevent the stacking effect that often leads to hypoglycemia.

Order Basal Insulin Therapy

Most hyperglycemic patients should receive basal insulin therapy in the hospital. Basal insulin can be an intermediate-acting insulin used twice daily or a long-acting insulin used once daily. Long-acting insulin may be administered in the morning or at bedtime. The dose of basal insulin can be decided on the basis of preadmission insulin needs or current insulin needs if on IV insulin infusion or body weight. In a patient with good glycemic control on insulin at home, total daily dose of insulin may be divided into 50% as basal insulin and 50% as the nutritional insulin need. In general, 80% of the preadmission basal insulin need is an appropriate starting dose. However, full dose or even a higher dose may be used if the admission HbA1c was high. In a patient coming off an insulin drip, insulin infusion rates in the last few hours may guide the basal insulin dose. However, if no information is available, weight-based basal insulin dose starting at 0.25 unit/kg is appropriate.

Order Nutritional Insulin Therapy

Once a patient starts receiving nutrition, insulin coverage is needed. Nutritional insulin coverage depends on the type of nutrition and it should be customized for each patient. If the patient is on an insulin infusion protocol, insulin infusion rates may be adjusted to cover all the nutritional insulin needs. For parenteral nutrition, regular insulin may be added to the IV nutrition. However, mostly the patients are switched to subcutaneous insulin when they start receiving enteral nutrition. In a patient eating regular meals, nutritional insulin doses may be assessed from the total daily dose of insulin and given as three equal premeal doses of a short-acting insulin. Nutritional insulin should be held if a meal is missed. It may be administered after a meal if oral intake is unreliable and reduced in proportion to the food intake. In a patient unable to eat regular meals but able to ingest semisolids or liquids, rapid-acting insulin is given before each meal. In a patient receiving tube feeds, rapid-acting insulin every 4 h or regular insulin every 6 h should be used during the duration of tube feeds. Often a much higher nutritional insulin coverage is needed with tube feeds than with regular meals. In a patient on bolus tube feeds, a rapid-acting insulin dose at the time of each bolus of tube feed should be ordered.

Order Hypoglycemia Protocol

All patients on insulin should have an order for hypoglycemia protocol. Treatment for hypoglycemia should start at BG level <70 mg/dL. Any low BG value should be confirmed by sending a stat plasma glucose test unless the patient is symptomatic in which case treatment should be administered immediately. If patients are able to eat, give 4 ounces of juice, non-diet soda, or 8 ounces of nonfat milk. If unable to eat but an IV line is in place, give dextrose 50% 1 ampule (25 g). If unable to take orally and no IV line is in place, give glucagon HCl 1 mg IM. Check BG every 15–30 min and repeat one of the three treatments till BG level is above 80 mg/dL.

Continue Insulin Pump if Patient Can Manage the Pump: Otherwise, Switch to Basal Bolus Insulin

Many patients with type 1 diabetes and some with type 2 diabetes may be using insulin pump before admission to hospital. Evaluate patients' proficiency with insulin pump, their clinical condition to manage their own pump, and the availability of pump supplies. If all conditions are ideal, i.e., the patient is well educated about insulin pump use and clinically (mentally and physically) able to take care of pump and can provide all their supplies for the pump, insulin pump can be continued as inpatient. Basal rates may need to be lowered (generally to about 80% of home dose) to prevent hypoglycemia. If the patient becomes unable to manage pump at any time during hospitalization, he/she should be switched to basal bolus insulin.

Review Blood Glucose (BG) Data Daily and Adjust Insulin Doses to Achieve Target BG Levels

It is important to review BG data at least once daily and adjust insulin doses to achieve target BG levels and to prevent hypoglycemia. Basal insulin should be adjusted to keep the fasting BG <140 mg/dL, and nutritional insulin should be adjusted to maintain all other BG levels in 100–180 range. Insulin doses should be increased by 10–20% at a time to produce a meaningful effect. A rapid increase in insulin dose may be appropriate depending on the clinical condition and BG levels. Any BG value <100 mg/dL in the previous 24 h should lead to a decrease in insulin dose to prevent hypoglycemia. Any BG <70 mg/dL or symptomatic hypoglycemia should lead to immediate reevaluation to prevent recurrence of hypoglycemia.

Evaluate Diabetes Treatment at Time of Discharge

Clinical condition may have changed during hospitalization necessitating changes to preadmission treatment for diabetes. Additionally, changes to diabetes treatment may be indicated due to poor preadmission diabetes control. In general, if HbA1c was <7% at time of admission, the patient should be discharged on the pre-hospitalization treatment. If HbA1s was 7–8%, adjust the pre-hospitalization treatment without making drastic changes to treatment. For example, doses of non-insulin agents or insulin may be increased or decreased, but avoid adding additional antidiabetic agents. An HbA1c >8% suggests that changes in treatment are needed but it depends on the glycemic goal for an individual patient. If a change in antidiabetic medications is made, the patient and the outpatient diabetes care provider should be informed of the change and the rationale for it, and a follow-up plan must be developed.

Follow-Up After Discharge

Discharge plan should include a timely follow-up visit for continued outpatient diabetes care. An appointment should be made for the patient to see their diabetes care providers within 7–30 days of discharge. Because glycemic control is expected to change after discharge, make sure that the patient is able to contact a diabetes care provider in case of high or low blood glucose levels.

Suggested Reading

American Diabetes Association. 14. Diabetes care in the hospital. Diabetes Care. 2017;40(Suppl 1):S120–7.

Garg R, Hudson M, editors. Hyperglycemia in the hospital setting. New Delhi: JP Brothers; 2014.

Umpierrez GE, Hellman R, Korytkowski MT, Kosiborod M, Maynard GA, Montori VM, et al. Management of hyperglycemia in hospitalized patients in non-critical care setting: an endocrine society clinical practice guideline. J Clin Endocrinol Metabol. 2012;97(1):16–38.

Hypoglycemia in Patients with Diabetes

23

Margo Hudson

Contents

M. Hudson (✉)
Brigham and Women's Hospital, Department of Endocrinology,
Hypertension and Diabetes, Boston, MA, USA
e-mail: mhudson@partners.org

© Springer Nature Switzerland AG 2020
R. K. Garg et al. (eds.), *Handbook of Inpatient Endocrinology*,
https://doi.org/10.1007/978-3-030-38976-5_23

Questions to Ask When a Patient with Diabetes Has Hypoglycemia in the Hospital

- Has the patient received insulin or sulfonylurea agent to cause hypoglycemia?
- Does the patient have an underlying condition predisposing to hypoglycemia such as renal or hepatic failure or advanced age?
- Was the insulin dose weight based or home dose?
- Are eating habits different in the hospital compared to home?
- Was prandial insulin mismatched to meal time or meal size?
- Were continuous tube feedings or TPN held or decreased?
- Was correctional insulin "stacked"?
- Were glucose checks done at correct times?
- Has there been a decrease in medications that cause hyperglycemia such as glucocorticoids or vasopressors?
- Does the hospital have systems in place to help detect, treat, and prevent hypoglycemia?

Defining Hypoglycemia in the Inpatient Setting

Inpatient hypoglycemia has previously been defined as any glucose <70 mg/dl (3.9 mmol/l) and severe hypoglycemia as glucose <40 mg/dl (2.2 mmol/l) independent of symptoms. However, as of 2017, the American Diabetes Association has modified the definition which now applies to inpatients and outpatients. Level 1 hypoglycemia is any glucose ≤70 mg/dL which is sufficiently low to warrant acute treatment with fast-acting carbohydrate as well as to adjust therapy to prevent in the future. Level 2 hypoglycemia is any level <54 mg/dL (3.0 mmol/l) which is sufficiently low to be considered serious and clinically important. Level 3 hypoglycemia is any glucose low enough to cause severe cognitive impairment which requires external assistance.

Detecting Hypoglycemia

Frequent glucose monitoring is required to detect hypoglycemia with use of insulin. Point of care (POC) testing provides immediate actionable results. Glucose values obtained with venous blood draws sent to the lab are generally less helpful than POC because of the significant time delay for resulting as well as a tendency for glucose levels to decrease in the tube unless sodium fluoride has been added to inhibit glycolysis. However, some medical conditions such as extremes of hematocrit and periph- eral ischemia may render POC testing less accurate and require venous draws. With IV insulin protocols, monitoring should be done at least every 1–2 h. With subcutaneous insulin, monitoring is usually at least four times a day: at meals and bedtime when patients are eating and every 6 h when they are NPO. In the inpa- tient setting, it is important to remember that patients may not manifest usual symptoms of hypoglycemia because of concomi- tant use of drugs that mask symptoms or diminished cognition from underlying medical conditions, so vigilance is important in detecting hypoglycemia.

Frequency of Hypoglycemia in Patients Treated with Insulin

Rates of hypoglycemia vary by severity of underlying condition (critical or noncritical), type of glycemic treatment (intravenous insulin or basal-bolus insulin or sliding scale alone), and target glucose range. In the Normoglycemia in Intensive Care Evaluation-Survival Using Glucose Algorithm Regulation (NICE- SUGAR) study, patients in the ICU were randomized to IV insu- lin targeting glucose of 80–110 mg/dl or 140–180 mg/dl. Nearly 7% of the patients with the lower glucose targets had at least one episode of BG below 40 mg/dl which was significantly greater than the less than 1% rate in the patients in the higher target range. In another study on a general surgical ward, patients with diabetes were randomized to basal-bolus insulin or sliding scale alone with glucose target ranges of 100–140 mg/dl in both groups. In the basal-bolus group, the mean glucose was 145 mg/dl, and in the sliding-scale-alone group, the mean glucose was 175 mg/dl. Incidence of glucose <70 mg/dl was 23% in the basal-bolus group and 4.7% in the sliding scale group. And, a third study looking at insulin dosing found that rates of hypoglycemia are greater with total daily doses of insulin exceeding 0.6 units/kg/day compared to lower doses. The implication of these studies is not to use sliding scale alone rather than basal-bolus or IV insulin but rather to use basal-bolus therapy or IV insulin with appropriate targets and methods for dose calculation. In order to reduce potential for hypoglycemia, most professional society guidelines suggest glucose target goals should be fasting 100–140 mg/dL, premeal <140 mg/dL, and random <180 mg/dL on the general medical ward and 140–180 mg/dl in the ICU setting.

Deleterious Effects of Hypoglycemia

Hypoglycemia in the inpatient setting is strongly associated with higher mortality. In a review of general ward patients with diabetes, each day with any BG <50 mg/dl was associated with an 85% increase in inpatient death, 65% increase in 1-year mortality, and 2.5 extra days of hospitalization. In another retrospective study, inpatients on insulin with an episode of hypoglycemia (BG <50 mg/dl) had an in-hospital mortality rate of 20.3% compared to 4.5% mortality rate in insulin-treated patients without hypoglycemia. In the NICE-SUGAR study, ICU patients on the lower target insulin drip protocol who had severe hypoglycemia (BG <40) had 79% higher mortality than patients on the same insulin drip protocol who did not experience hypoglycemia. In the subset of patients with diabetes, moderate hypoglycemia was associated with 58% higher mortality and severe hypoglycemia with 85% higher mortality than patients with diabetes who did not have hypoglycemia. Whether hypoglycemia is the driver of higher mortality or a marker of poor health, it is clear that it should be avoided if possible.

Identifying Patients Most at Risk for Hypoglycemia

Patients admitted to the hospital often have multiple medical problems. The elderly and patients with renal or hepatic failure are at high risk for hypoglycemia because of decreased gluconeogenesis as well as decreased insulin metabolism. Another risk

Table 23.1 High-risk situations for hypoglycemia

1. Change in nutrition
(a) Holding TPN, tube feeds, or sudden NPO status
(b) Patient off floor at meal time
2. Drop in steroid dose
3. Patients who are on pressors and iv insulin together who then have pressors decreased
4. Acute kidney or liver injury
5. Stress hyperglycemia treated with insulin when stress resolves

group is patients with unusually high outpatient insulin doses (over 1 unit/kg/day total daily dose) which may indicate either noncompliance or excess caloric intake, both of which will be corrected in the hospital, and therefore giving 80% of the usual outpatient dose or recalculating with standard weight-based dosing may be prudent.

Common inpatient situations that lead to an acute drop in insulin requirements are listed in Table 23.1. Change in nutrition is responsible for many episodes of hypoglycemia. Patients with insulin "on board" and who are on TPN or enteral tube feeds who have the feedings held or decreased or patients who are eating and are made NPO or do not eat a complete meal are particularly vulnerable. Other common high-risk scenarios include patients on high-dose steroids who have the steroid dose dropped, patients on high insulin infusion rates due to vasopressors who have them tapered, and patients who develop acute renal, hepatic, or adrenal failure. Patients who are actually improving such as patients with sepsis or MI and secondary acute hyperglycemia (stress hyperglycemia) will see glucose levels drop and insulin requirements decrease. Hypoglycemia should be anticipated in all these situations and insulin doses dropped preemptively to prevent hypoglycemia.

When subcutaneous insulin has already been given, short-term IV glucose infusion may be necessary to avoid hypoglycemia. For patients on continuous tube feeds, for example, that are abruptly discontinued (e.g., patient pulls out NG tube), D5W at the rate of the tube feeds or D10 at half the rate of the tube feeds will usually be adequate to avoid short-term hypoglycemia until beyond the period of active insulin action or the tube feeds can be restored. Communication between nursing and providers is essential to manage these situations that often are unpredictable.

Insulin Action

Medications that may contribute to hypoglycemia in the inpatient setting include drugs in the sulfonylurea class (glyburide, glipizide, glimepiride in the United States), meglitinides (usually repaglinide), and all insulins. In general, use of oral agents is discouraged in the hospital because of unpredictable and prolonged action, especially in the setting of hepatic or renal dysfunction or interruption of nutritional patterns.

Insulin is the most widely used medication to treat hyperglycemia in the inpatient setting because the many types of insulin offer a wide range of available action profiles to allow greater flexibility in dosing. However, insulin is also responsible for medication-induced hypoglycemia because of its narrow therapeutic window. Insulin action profiles are shown in Table 23.2. Patients are most at risk for hypoglycemia at the peak action of the insulin. When two types of insulin are used, hypoglycemic potential will be additive. Premixed insulin is not recommended in the hospital setting because the faster-acting and longer-acting components cannot be individually adjusted. When regular insulin is given IV either as a bolus or as a continuous drip, the impact is immediate and action can persist for up to an hour after the dose.

Initial Dosing of Insulin to Avoid Hypoglycemia

In patients naive to insulin who are admitted to the hospital, a framework for prescribing insulin is critical to assist in meeting glucose targets and avoid hypoglycemia. Weight; age; renal, hepatic, and pancreatic functions; and steroid use all impact insulin requirements. Generally insulin is prescribed using a combination of intermediate- or long-acting insulin (basal) with short- or

Table 23.2 Insulin action profiles (subcutaneously)

Type of insulin	Name	Onset	Peak	Duration
Rapid acting	Aspart (Novolog) Lispro (Humalog) Glulisine (Apidra)	5–15 min	1–2 h	4–6 h
Short acting	Regular (Humulin R, Novolin R)	30–60 min	2–4 h	6–10 h
Intermediate acting	NPH (Humulin N, Novolin N) U-500 regular insulin (only for use in insulin-resistant patients)	2–4 h 30–60 min	6–12 h 2–4 h	12–18 h 6–8 h
Long acting	Glargine (Lantus) Detemir (Levemir)	2–4 h	None	22–24 h 17–24 h
	Glargine (Toujeo) Degludec (Tresiba)	6 h 1 h	None None	22–36 h 42 h
Premixed insulin	NPH/regular (Humulin 70/30, Novolin 70/30)	30–60 min	2–12 h	12–18 h
	Lispro protamine/lispro (Humalog 75/25, Humalog 50/50)	5–15 min	1–2 h	12–18 h
	Aspart protamine/aspart (Novolog 70/30)	5–15 min	1–2 h	12–18 h

rapid-acting insulin (nutritional and correctional). The schema in Fig. 23.1 is a handy way to calculate the doses. For patients on TF or glucocorticoid treatment, consider using 60% of TDD as nutritional component rather than 50%.

Correctional insulin (sliding scale) can be prescribed based on the calculated total daily dose so that if TDD is less than or equal to 40 units, use a correctional scale of 1 unit rapid-acting or short-acting insulin for every 50 mg/dl above goal. For TDD over 40 units a day, consider using 1 unit for every 25 mg/dl above goal. Correctional insulin is generally given with a rapid-acting insulin analog before meals and before bed in patients who are eating and with regular human insulin every 6 h in patients who are on continuous feedings, TPN, or NPO. Outside of hyperglycemic emergencies, correctional insulin should not be given more frequently than this to avoid hypoglycemia from overlapping the

a

Baseline weight-based TDD Estimate	0.5 unit/kg/day, adjust by factors listed below
Age > 70 years	–0.1 unit/kg/day
Renal insufficiency (eGFR < 45)	–0.1 unit/kg/day
Advanced Cirrhosis	–0.1 unit/kg/day
Pancreatic deficiency (chronic pancreatitis, cystic fibrosis, s/p pancreatectomy)	–0.1 unit/kg/day
HbA1c >10%	+0.1 unit/kg/day
Currently on glucocorticoids with equivalent of prednisone 40 mg/day or greater	+0.1 unit/kg/day
FINAL TDD estimate	?

b

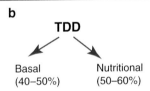

TDD

Basal (40–50%)   Nutritional (50–60%)

Example: 60 kg patient with TDD estimate 0.5 unit/kg/day
0.5 X 60 = 30 units TDD with 50% basal and 50% nutritional
30÷2=15 units basal and 15 units prandial (5 units AC)

Fig. 23.1 (**a**) *Step 1*: initiation of insulin and determination of total daily dose (TDD). *Use weight or if patients on insulin as outpatient consider 80% of home dose, but not to exceed 1 unit/kg TDD* (**b**) *Step 2*: Components of insulin program: *basal, nutritional, correctional.* (Reprinted from Hudson M.S., Palermo N.E. Diabetes in Older Adults, pp. 1–18, In: Rosenthal R., Zenilman M., Katlic M. (eds) Principles and Practice of Geriatric Surgery, © 2017, with permission from Springer Nature. See Suggested Readings)

actions of repeated doses, a phenomenon known as "stacking." Some institutions give only "half" scale for bedtime correctional insulin to avoid potential for overnight hypoglycemia.

What to Do When Hypoglycemia Occurs

All hospitals should have protocols in place for managing acute hypoglycemia both on the general wards and in the ICU. Generally, treatment should be started in the hospital when glucose falls below 70 mg/dl. If possible, patients should be treated orally. A nursing protocol should be in place for treatment (Fig. 23.2).

The art of managing hypoglycemia is to determine which insulin dose may be responsible for an episode of hypoglycemia and how much it should be reduced. Knowing the insulin action profile (see Table 23.2) is helpful. Generally the early morning glucose is the best reflection of the action of basal insulin, but this may not be the case if the patient is receiving rapid-acting insulin late at night (nighttime correctional scales) or overnight (e.g., with continuous enteral nutrition). Premeal or pre-bed hypoglycemia may reflect the rapid-acting insulin given with the previous meal.

If the hypoglycemia is associated with a significant change in medical condition (stopping steroids, e.g., or acute renal failure), dose adjustments in the range of 30–50% may be necessary. However, if the patient is otherwise clinically stable, a simple calculation for adjusting insulin is to decrease the TDD of insulin by

Treatment of Hypoglycemia

1. Give 15 g of sugar (no artificial sweetners) as $^1/_2$ cup of fruit juice **or** 1 cup skim **or** 3 packs of sugar in water **or** 3 – 4 commercial glucose tablets (4–5 g glucose each).

2. Wait 15 min and re-test blood sugar. Retreat until glucose is at least over 70 mg/dl.

3. If the patient is unable to take orally for any reason (loss of consciousness, aspiration risk, etc.) glucose should be given IV generally 12.5–25 g of dextrose as D50 IV push.

4. If patient does not have an adequate IV to handle D50W push, then glucagon 1 mg IV or IM can be given.

Fig. 23.2   Treatment of hypoglycemia

10% for glucose values running 70–99 mg/dl and to decrease the TDD by 20% for any glucose value below 70 mg/dl.

Hospital Surveillance and Reporting: Glucometrics

Hospitals should have in place quality improvement programs to monitor glucose values generally and episodes of hypoglycemia specifically so that areas with recurrent problems can be identified and causes addressed. The Society for Hospital Medicine has developed a national Glucose Control Mentored Implementation Program that hospitals can join to report their glucose values. The hospital can then be benchmarked against other institutions for metrics such as days with any glucose below 70 mg/dl. In this way, the institution can assess performance on a national level and hopefully find ways to improve patient care. For more information, go to http://dev.hospitalmedicine.org/Web/Quality_Innovation/Implementation_Toolkits/Glycemic_Control/Web/Quality___Innovation/Implementation_Toolkit/Glycemic/Track_Performance/Introducing_Glucometrics.aspx

Beyond Basal-Bolus Insulin: Glucose Control Without Hypoglycemia

Because of concern for hypoglycemia and its potentially devastating consequences, improvements on current basal-bolus treatment recommendations are being actively studied. A trial comparing basal-bolus insulin to basal plus correctional insulin (i.e., no scheduled mealtime insulin) showed similar average glucose values but less moderate hypoglycemia (<70 mg/dl) in the basal plus correctional treatment group. Other trials have looked at using DPP-4 inhibitors or GLP-1 receptor agonist agents in the inpatient setting, but these have not received general acceptance at this time.

Suggested Reading

American Diabetes Association. Diabetes care in the hospital. Diabetes Care. 2017a;40(Suppl 1):S120–7.

American Diabetes Association. Glycemic targets. Sec 6. In Standards of medical care in diabetes–2017. Diabetes Care. 2017b;40(Suppl. 1): S48–56.

Garg R, Hurwitz S, Turchin A, Trivedi A. Hypoglycemia, with or without insulin therapy, is associated with increased mortality among hospitalized patients. Diabetes Care. 2013;36(5):1107–10.

Hudson MS, Palermo NE. Diabetes in older adults. In: Rosenthal R, Zenilman M, Katlic M, editors. Principles and practice of geriatric surgery. Cham: Springer; 2017. p. 1–18.

NICE-SUGAR Study Investigators, Finfer S, Chittock DR, Su SY, Blair D, Foster D, et al. Intensive versus conventional glucose control in critically ill patients. N Engl J Med. 2009;360(13):1283–97.

Rubin DJ, Rybin D, Doros G, McDonnell ME. Weight-based, insulin dose-related hypoglycemia in hospitalized patients with diabetes. Diabetes Care. 2011;34(8):1723–8.

Society of Hospital Medicine. Quality & innovation. External sources & benchmarking/glycemic control implementation toolkit 2017 https://www.hospitalmedicine.org/Web/Quality_Innovation/Implementation_Toolkits/Glycemic_Control/Web/Quality___Innovation/Implementation_Toolkit/Glycemic/Track_Performance/external_sources_benchmarking.aspx.

Turchin A, Matheny ME, Shubina M, Scanlon JV, Greenwood B, Pendergrass ML. Hypoglycemia and clinical outcomes in patients with diabetes hospitalized in the general ward. Diabetes Care. 2009;32(7):1153–7.

Umpierrez GE, Smiley D, Jacobs S, Peng L, Temponi A, Mulligan P, Umpierrez D, et al. Randomized study of basal-bolus insulin therapy in the inpatient management of patients with type 2 diabetes undergoing general surgery (RABBIT 2 surgery). Diabetes Care. 2011;34(2):256–61.

Umpierrez GE, Smiley D, Hermayer K, Khan A, Olson DE, Newton C, et al. Randomized study comparing a Basal-bolus with a basal plus correction insulin regimen for the hospital management of medical and surgical patients with type 2 diabetes: basal plus trial. Diabetes Care. 2013;36(8):2169–74.

Hypoglycemia in Patients Without Diabetes

24

Rajesh K. Garg

Contents

R. K. Garg (✉)
Division of Endocrinology, Diabetes and Metabolism,
University of Miami Miller School of Medicine, Coral Gables, FL, USA
e-mail: rgarg@miami.edu

© Springer Nature Switzerland AG 2020
R. K. Garg et al. (eds.), *Handbook of Inpatient Endocrinology*,
https://doi.org/10.1007/978-3-030-38976-5_24

Diagnosis of Hypoglycemia in Patients Without Major Acute or Chronic Illness

Symptoms and signs of hypoglycemia are often nonspecific. Therefore, Whipple's triad must be satisfied to make a diagnosis of hypoglycemia. Whipple's triad includes low blood glucose levels, the presence of symptoms or signs of hypoglycemia at the time of low blood glucose levels, and recovery from symptoms or signs by raising blood glucose levels.

Diagnosis in Patients with Major Illness

Sick patients may not feel symptoms or signs of hypoglycemia. Therefore, any blood glucose <55 mg/dL needs evaluation in a sick person. Spontaneous hypoglycemia in a sick person is often not caused by hyperinsulinemia. Both insulin-mediated and non-insulin-mediated hypoglycemia in the hospital setting are associated with high mortality.

Symptoms and Signs of Hypoglycemia

Symptoms and signs of hypoglycemia can be divided into autonomic or neuroglycopenic. Autonomic symptoms and signs including hunger, palpitation, anxiety, tachycardia, tremor, pallor, and diaphoresis appear early as the blood glucose levels start going down. Neuroglycopenic symptoms and signs including behavioral changes, confusion, loss of consciousness, and seizures appear later and at much lower blood glucose levels. However, in patients getting frequent hypoglycemic episodes, autonomic symptoms and signs may be suppressed, and as a result they may present with neuroglycopenic symptoms.

Causes of Hypoglycemia

Medications

The most common medications that cause hypoglycemia are insulin or insulin secretagogues and alcohol. However, the list of drugs associated with hypoglycemia is long and ever growing. Check all current medications that a patient is taking that may cause hypoglycemia. However, the evidence regarding association between most drugs and hypoglycemia is rather weak. Therefore, in many cases, diagnosis of drug-induced hypoglycemia can only be made after excluding other causes. More often, drugs are a contributing factor to hypoglycemia caused by another major problem, like organ system failure.

Organ System Failure Like Cardiac, Renal, or Liver Failure

The liver is the main glucogenic organ with the kidney contributing to gluconeogenesis to some extent. Therefore, hypoglycemia is common in the presence of liver failure, and the risk of hypoglycemia increases in the presence of renal failure. Severe heart failure can cause hypoglycemia due to inanition and liver congestion.

Sepsis and Adrenal or Pituitary Insufficiency Are All Associated with Hypoglycemia

Major illness is evident in this setting. A high index of suspicion and targeted testing are needed to rule in adrenal and pituitary insufficiency.

Non-islet Cell Tumors

Tumors associated with hypoglycemic are mostly large mesen-chymal tumors that secrete IGF-II. In these cases, IGF-II level or its ratio to IGF-I is increased. However, a few reports of IGF-1 secreting tumors leading to hypoglycemia have also been published.

Antibody-Induced Hypoglycemia

Insulin antibodies can bind endogenous insulin and release it in large amounts periodically to cause hypoglycemia. Antibodies may also directly bind to insulin receptors and cause hypoglyce-mia. In the presence of antibody-induced hypoglycemia, insulin levels are often reported extremely high (>100 mU/L) due to the antibodies interfering with the insulin assay. C-peptide and proin-sulin levels can be high, normal, or low.

Endogenous Insulin Production

Insulinoma- and non-insulinoma-related hyperinsulinemia are rare but important causes of hypoglycemia. Insulinomas are often small, single, benign tumors with very low recurrence rate after resection. However, they may also occur as part of the MEN-1 syndrome where they can be multiple and have a high recurrence rate. Non-insulinoma-related hyperinsulinemia has been described most often after bariatric surgery. It is due to diffuse islet hypertrophy, sometimes with hyperplasia, also called as nesidio-blastosis. No single lesion can be identified in these cases, making treatment very difficult. Endogenous insulin secretion due to drugs like sulfonylureas or meglitinides must be ruled out before making a diagnosis of insulinoma- and non-insulinoma-related hyperinsulinemia.

Pseudohypoglycemia

Pseudohypoglycemia can happen in conditions with increased number of red or white blood cells. It may also happen when the blood sample is collected in a tube without an inhibitor of glycolysis or when the processing of blood sample for glucose measurement is delayed.

Laboratory Investigations for Hypoglycemia

Laboratory investigations for hypoglycemia are necessary unless there is a clear cause of hypoglycemia, in which case it will resolve after the cause is addressed (Table 24.1). Investigations for the cause of hypoglycemia must be performed at the time of the condition. Induction of hypoglycemia may be necessary if the episodes of spontaneous hypoglycemia are infrequent. Blood glucose from finger-stick blood samples is appropriate for monitoring while waiting for a symptomatic episode of hypoglycemia. However, venous blood samples for the following laboratory tests should be collected at the time of hypoglycemia: glucose, insulin, C-peptide, proinsulin, beta-hydroxybutyrate, and sulfonylureas. After collecting blood, patient should receive an IV injection of 1.0 mg glucagon, and then finger-stick and plasma glucose should be measured at 10, 20, and 30 min after the injection.

Prolonged Fasting Test

A prolonged fasting test is indicated when the patient complains of fasting hypoglycemia, but it is hard to observe an episode of spontaneous hypoglycemia. A prolonged fast test can take up to 72 h to be diagnostic. A sufficient amount of noncaloric, non-caffeinated beverages may be administered during the test in order to prevent dehydration. Although it can be started at any

Table 24.1 Differential diagnosis of spontaneous hypoglycemia

Diagnosis	Laboratory tests	Comment
Endogenous insulin production: insulinoma and diffuse islet cell hyperplasia	High insulin, C-peptide, and proinsulin Low beta-hydroxybutyrate Response to glucagon Absence of insulin secretagogue drugs	Prolonged fasting may be required to induce hypoglycemia
Exogenous insulin	High insulin Low C-peptide and proinsulin Low beta-hydroxybutyrate Response to glucagon Absence of insulin secretagogue drugs	Detailed history may reveal exogenous insulin use
Drug induced: sulfonylurea-like drugs	High insulin, C-peptide, and proinsulin Low beta-hydroxybutyrate Response to glucagon Presence of insulin secretagogue drugs	Detailed history including examination of all drugs and supplements is important
Non-islet tumors: producing IGF-II	Low insulin, C-peptide, and proinsulin Low beta-hydroxybutyrate Response to glucagon Absence of insulin secretagogue drugs High IGF-II levels	Presence of tumor may be obvious
Non-insulin- or insulin-like factor-related condition: organ system failure, endocrine deficiencies	Low insulin, C-peptide, and proinsulin High beta-hydroxybutyrate No response to glucagon Absence of insulin secretagogue drugs	Presence of obvious severe acute or chronic illness
Antibody mediated	Very high insulin levels High or low C-peptide and proinsulin Low beta-hydroxybutyrate Response to glucagon Absence of insulin secretagogue drugs	Blood glucose levels highly variable. Other autoimmune conditions may be present

time of the day in a patient admitted to hospital, it is best that the prolonged fast test be started in the morning because the majority of patients with significant underlying pathology are likely to become hypoglycemic within the first 8 h and appropriate testing would be possible before the night shift when access to staff and other resources may be limited. However, if hypoglycemia does not develop within 8 h, fasting should continue until the time of symptomatic hypoglycemia or up to 72 h before ending the fast. Patients should be closely monitored for signs and symptoms including mental status checks along with finger-stick blood glucose determinations. Low blood glucose values should be confirmed by laboratory plasma glucose determination. The prolonged fast test should be ended when the patient is symptomatic with plasma glucose <55 mg/dL or the plasma glucose is <45 mg/dL even without symptoms or 72 h have elapsed. Laboratory investigations described in previous section should be obtained at this point before ending the prolonged fast test.

Mixed Meal Test

If hypoglycemia symptoms occur postprandially, a mixed meal test may be able to induce hypoglycemia and allow investigation at the time of hypoglycemia. In general, the meal should be similar to the one that causes spontaneous hypoglycemia. However, if this not practical, a liquid nutritional formula may be used. The test should be conducted in the morning after an overnight fast. Blood glucose should be monitored every 30 min for 4 h. Blood glucose criteria for ending the test are similar to those for the prolonged fast test.

Differentiating Insulin-Mediated Versus Non-insulin-Mediated Hypoglycemia

Diagnosis of endogenous hyperinsulinemia depends on demonstrating high insulin, high C-peptide, high proinsulin, low beta-hydroxybutyrate, and absence of sulfonylureas and meglitinides at the time of hypoglycemia. Because hypoglycemia should normally suppress insulin and C-peptide levels, a plasma insulin level of ≥3.0 microU/ml and a C-peptide level of ≥0.6 ng/ml in the presence of hypoglycemia are considered abnormal. A proinsulin level of ≥5.0 pmol/L is also highly suggestive of hyperinsulinism due to insulinoma. If insulin levels are high in the absence of high C-peptide or proinsulin levels, exogenous insulin-induced hypoglycemia should be suspected. Insulin effectively suppresses ketone production, and a beta-hydroxybutyrate level of ≤2.7 mmol/L is indicative of an increased insulin-like effect. An increase in plasma glucose of at least 25 mg/dl after intravenous glucagon also indicates mediation of the hypoglycemia by insulin-like effect. Therefore, low beta-hydroxybutyrate and adequate response to glucagon in the absence of high levels of insulin suggest the presence of IGF. Insulin secretagogue drugs like sulfonylureas and meglitinides cause hypoglycemia, and their presence should be ruled out before making a diagnosis of insulinoma or non-insulinoma hyperinsulinism. Non-insulin-mediated hypoglycemia will be associated with low insulin, low C-peptide, low proinsulin, high beta-hydroxybutyrate, and inadequate response to glucagon. In severely hypoglycemic patients, glucose requirement >8 mg/kg/min (normal 4–6 mg/kg min) to maintain normoglycemia suggests hypoglycemia likely due to excess of insulin or insulin-like growth factor secretion.

Imaging Studies for Insulinoma

Imaging for insulinoma should be ordered only when the biochemical diagnosis has been definitively made. The majority of insulinomas are <2 cm in size. Computed tomography or MRI can identify about 80% of insulinomas. When a lesion is not seen on CT scan or MRI scan, endoscopic pancreatic ultrasonography should be the next modality of imaging because it will detect most remaining insulinomas. Sometimes, an octreotide scan or gallium dotatate PET/CT scan may be ordered. When an insulinoma is not visible on any of the imaging studies, hepatic venous sampling after selective arterial calcium injections may be required. In this method, calcium gluconate is sequentially injected into the splenic, gastroduodenal, and superior mesenteric arteries, and a twofold increase in insulin levels in the hepatic vein will localize the source of excess insulin to the tail of the pancreas, body of the pancreas, or head of the pancreas. Imaging using 18-FDG PET is of no proven value at this time. However, it may be useful in localization of the cause of non-insulin-mediated tumorigenic hypoglycemia.

Treatment of Hypoglycemia

Treatment of hypoglycemia depends on the cause of hypoglycemia, and it may be achieved by treatment of the underlying cause or surgical removal of the cause, e.g., discontinuing the offending drug, hormonal replacement, treating sepsis, or removing an islet cell tumor. In the short term, treatment of hypoglycemia or its prevention is important. Frequent oral feeding or intravenous glucose or glucagon may be needed. Most cases of insulinoma are cured after surgery. However, some patients with malignant insulinoma- or non-insulinoma-mediated hyperinsulinism may need chronic treatment with diazoxide or octreotide or parenteral nutrition. Rare patients with nesidioblastosis may require partial or complete pancreatectomy to relieve hypoglycemia. The patient with an IGF-producing malignant tumor may also be difficult to treat. Patients with antibody-induced hypoglycemia may respond to glucocorticoids or immunosuppressive treatment.

Suggested Reading

Cryer PE, Axelrod L, Grossman AB, Heller SR, Montori VM, Seaquist ER, Service FJ, Endocrine Society. Evaluation and management of adult hypoglycemic disorders: an Endocrine Society Clinical Practice Guideline. J Clin Endocrinol Metabol. 2009;94(3):709–28.

Garg R, Hurwitz S, Turchin A, Trivedi A. Hypoglycemia, with or without insulin therapy, is associated with increased mortality among hospitalized patients. Diabetes Care. 2013;36(5):1107–10.

Martens P, Tits J. Approach to the patient with spontaneous hypoglycemia. Eur J Intern Med. 2014;25(5):415–21.

Salehi M, Vella A, McLaughlin T, Patti ME. Hypoglycemia after gastric bypass surgery: current concepts and controversies. J Clin Endocrinol Metabol. 2018;103(8):2815–26.

Diabetic Ketoacidosis and Hyperosmolar Hyperglycemic State

25

Daniela V. Pirela and Rajesh K. Garg

Contents

D. V. Pirela
Jackson Memorial Hospital/University of Miami Hospital,
Division of Endocrinology, Diabetes and Metabolism, Miami, FL, USA

R. K. Garg (✉)
Division of Endocrinology, Diabetes and Metabolism,
University of Miami Miller School of Medicine, Coral Gables, FL, USA
e-mail: rgarg@miami.edu

© Springer Nature Switzerland AG 2020
R. K. Garg et al. (eds.), *Handbook of Inpatient Endocrinology*,
https://doi.org/10.1007/978-3-030-38976-5_25

Epidemiology

According to the CDC data, there were 207,000 emergency department visits for hyperglycemic crisis in the year 2014. This amounts to 9.5 visits per 1000 persons with diabetes for DKA or HHS. However, these two entities represent an extreme on the spectrum of avoidable hyperglycemic emergencies in patients with diabetes; majority of patients are admitted with hyperglycemia along with another illness. Females, adolescents, ethnic minorities, and patients with high A1c are at higher risk of DKA or HHS.

The incidence of DKA has gone up, at least 6% annually from 2009 to 2014 in all age groups. Although DKA is considered pathognomonic of type 1 diabetes, at least one-third of the DKA cases occur in patients with type 2 diabetes. HHS is less common and represents less than 1% of all diabetes-related admissions. Although generally seen in adults with type 2 diabetes, HHS is becoming more frequent among children and young adults.

DKA causes almost 50% of all deaths in patients with type 1 diabetes under the age of 24 years. Inpatient DKA mortality is less than 1%, while for HHS, mortality is as high as 16%. Even though the mortality risk has declined, mortality and morbidity related to acute hyperglycemic emergencies remain high, and the health-care costs remain substantial, especially taking into account the increase in incidence.

Diagnosis of DKA

Signs and Symptoms

Evolution of DKA is rather acute. Patients often complain of fatigue and osmotic symptoms like polyuria and polydipsia. Abdominal pain, nausea, and vomiting are present in up to two-thirds of patients. The severity of symptoms depends on multiple factors including the severity of acidosis, dehydration, and age of the patient. Neurologic symptoms such as lethargy and stupor develop in half of patients when serum osmolarity reaches 320 mOsmol/kg; loss of consciousness occurs in less than 25% of patients. Presence of altered mental status and a serum osmolarity less than 320 should prompt additional neurologic workup. Abdominal pain is more common in younger patients and seems to be related to the severity of the metabolic acidosis, which interferes with gastric emptying. In the absence of metabolic acidosis or if abdominal pain persists despite resolution of DKA, pancreatitis and other gastrointestinal disorders should be considered. Dry mucosa, decreased skin turgor, and low jugular venous pressure can be appreciated in most of the patients due to dehydration. The presence of tachycardia and hypotension correlates with the degree of dehydration. Patients may have a fruity odor to their breath due to the exhaled ketones as well as deep hyperventilation (Kussmaul respirations).

Laboratory Tests

To make a diagnosis of DKA, the triad of hyperglycemia above 250 mg/dL, ketonemia, and metabolic acidosis with elevated anion gap should be present. Plasma glucose is usually between 350 and 500 mg/dL when the patient presents to the emergency department. Some patients with DKA may present with only mild elevations of blood glucose levels. This is known as euglycemic DKA; this can be seen in patients with prolonged starvation, alcohol intake, insufficient insulin dose, and pregnancy and in patients using SGLT-2 inhibitors that lead to glycosuria, blunting the elevation of blood glucose level.

Hyperglycemia is secondary to the deficit of effective insulin, the excess of counterregulatory hormones, and relative increase in insulin resistance. Insulin normally blocks ketogenesis by inhibiting lipolysis and the transport of free fatty acid derivatives into the mitochondrial matrix. Insulin deficiency leads to unrestrained lipolysis and mobilization of triglycerides and amino acids for energy use instead of glucose. Increased levels of serum free fatty acids are converted to ketones bodies and acids which are mainly acetoacetic acid and beta-hydroxybutyric acid, both strong organic acids. Hepatic gluconeogenesis is stimulated by glucagon excess and excess of other stress hormones, while alanine originated from muscle catabolism and glycerol from lipolysis provide the substrate.

The metabolic imbalance is characterized by a low bicarbonate level, usually less than 18 mEq/L, and the accumulation of keto acids in blood that cause a drop in the arterial pH to less than 7.3 with an elevation of the anion gap above 12. In DKA, keto acids become circulating unmeasured anions. In addition, lactic acid generated from tissue hypoxia contributes to unmeasured anions further increasing the anion gap. The anion gap is calculated by the following formula:

$$\text{Anion gap} = \left[\text{Sodium}\left(mEq\,/\,L\right) + \text{Potassium}\left(mEq\,/\,L\right) \right] \\ - \left[\text{Chloride}\left(mEq\,/\,L\right) + HCO_3 - \left(mEq\,/\,L\right) \right]$$

The nitroprusside test can detect ketones bodies, more specifically acetoacetate, in the urine. This test does not correlate with disease severity as it can be negative in severe ketosis when beta-hydroxybutyrate becomes the predominant ketone or when lactic acidosis coexists with the ketoacidosis interfering with the measurement of the acetoacetate. Serum ketone levels usually are done when urine ketone test is positive; however, due to the high false-negative and false-positive urine nitroprusside tests, direct measurement of serum beta-hydroxybutyrate is preferred.

Hyperglycemia may cause non-hypotonic hyponatremia. Glucose is an osmotically active substance. Therefore, in the presence of hyperglycemia, increased plasma osmolality induces water movement to the extracellular space leading to reduction of serum sodium levels which is also called dilutional hyponatremia. Therefore, corrected serum sodium level should be used to calculate an accurate serum anion gap. To correct serum sodium level, add 1.6 mEq/L to the measured serum sodium for each 100 mg/dL of glucose greater than 100 mg/dL. A normal measured sodium level in the setting of hyperglycemic DKA is suggestive of profound hypovolemia. Serum bicarbonate is usually below 10 mmol/l and pH 6.8–7.3. Infrequently, the pH may not be significantly decreased due to compensatory hyperventilation, which will decrease the partial pressure of carbon dioxide.

There is an increased urinary loss of potassium due to the glucose osmotic diuresis and the excretion of potassium keto acid anion salts which lead to deficit of the total body potassium. The metabolic acidosis, hyperosmolarity, and insulin deficiency cause a shift of potassium from intracellular fluid to extracellular fluid. Therefore, the serum potassium concentration is usually normal or even elevated initially. Once insulin therapy is introduced, potassium shifts back into cells which rapidly lower the potassium concentration and may lead to severe hypokalemia.

At presentation, serum phosphate is usually normal or high because both insulin deficiency and metabolic acidosis cause a shift of phosphate out of the cells. However, there is a decreased phosphate intake and phosphaturia caused by osmotic diuresis that result in a net phosphate depletion. Thus, after volume and insulin replacement, hypophosphatemia ensues.

Diagnosis of HHS

Signs and Symptoms

Hyperosmolar hyperglycemic state (HHS) presentation has a less acute presentation than DKA. Symptoms of polyuria, polydipsia, and weight loss are more evident and often start several days or weeks before the hospital admission. Blurred vision and progressive decline in mental status are also evident.

Severe dehydration and high plasma osmolarity lead to mental obtundation and coma that are proportional to the degree and rate of the development of hyperosmolarity. Decreased skin turgor, dry oral mucosa, low jugular venous pressure, tachycardia, and hypotension are more evident in HHS compared to DKA. Rarely patients can develop abdominal pain.

Laboratory Tests

The serum glucose concentration is much higher, frequently exceeding 600 mg/dL, but can be higher than 1000 mg/dL in HHS. The endogenous insulin production is sufficient to suppress ketogenesis. Therefore, ketone levels remain within normal limits, which means the pH, the serum bicarbonate, and the anion gap stay normal as well. The glycosuria leads to severe dehydration and an effective plasma osmolarity typically above 320 mOsmol/kg. Hyponatremia is usually present through the same mechanism as in DKA and is sometimes more severe. Similar to DKA, the serum potassium concentration is usually normal, though in one-third of patients it is elevated up to 5.7 mEq/L on admission. After proper insulin therapy and fluid resuscitation, potassium shifts back into the cells uncovering the total body potassium deficit. Other laboratory results such as leukocytosis, increased BUN, and creatinine are proportional to the degree of hypovolemia.

Management

Most Common Causes to Rule Out

- Medication nonadherence.
- Infections. Obtain urine and blood cultures, chest radiograph, and other tests in selected cases.
- Pancreatitis. Obtain serum lipase and amylase when pancreatitis is clinically suspected. The result must be interpreted with caution because some increase in amylase can be associated with DKA itself.
- Tissue ischemia such as cardiac ischemia and cerebrovascular accidents. Obtain cardiac enzymes and electrocardiogram, and perform neurologic assessment.
- Concomitant medications. Look for medications that may have precipitated the acute hyperglycemic emergency including glucocorticoids, beta-blockers, thiazide diuretics, certain

chemotherapeutic agents, atypical antipsychotics, and SGLT2 inhibitors.

- Severe dehydration. Mainly bedridden and elderly patients are in danger of having compromised access to water; this is exacerbated by the altered thirst response in some of them. Newly diagnosed and even undiagnosed fragile patients, particularly residents of chronic care facilities, may be at risk of delayed recognition of hyperglycemic symptoms and severe dehydration. Administration of insulin, without initial proper fluid replacement, may accentuate hyperosmolality by moving water intracellularly which further aggravate vascular collapse, hypotension, and even death.

IV Fluids

Intravenous fluid is the mainstay of management of hyperglycemic crises. Fluids improve the clinical and metabolic status by decreasing serum glucose through urinary clearance by improving renal perfusion and by intravascular volume expansion. Isotonic saline is initially infused at 500–1000 ml/h for 2–4 h, followed by the infusion of 0.9% or 0.45% saline at 250–500 ml/h depending on the serum sodium level, the state of hydration, and the urine output. In general, 0.9% saline is continued in patients with low serum sodium, whereas patients with normal or elevated serum sodium or hyperosmolarity should receive 0.45% NaCl. Intravenous dextrose (5% or 10%) is added once the plasma glucose level is between 200 and 250 mg/dL, to allow continued insulin administration until ketonemia is controlled while avoiding hypoglycemia.

Insulin Therapy

Insulin is key component of treatment of DKA and HHS. In general, DKA resolution occurs between 10 and 18 h after initiation of therapy, while HHS resolution can take longer. Intravenous regular insulin has been the treatment of choice for the management of acute hyperglycemic emergencies, but the use of subcutaneous insulin for mild-to-moderate DKA is becoming more common. The time of resolution seems to be equivalent with either option, but the use of subcutaneous insulin mitigates the burden on the nursing staff. Insulin reduces hepatic gluconeogenesis and suppresses lipolysis and ketogenesis. Insulin therapy will shift extracellular potassium into the intracellular space. Therefore, to avoid severe hypokalemia, serum potassium should be more than 3.3 mEq/L when insulin therapy is started.

An intravenous bolus of regular insulin at a rate of 0.1 unit/kg followed by a continuous infusion at a rate of 0.1 U/kg/h (5–10 U/h) vs no bolus and infusion of insulin at a rate of 0.14 U/kg/h has shown similar outcomes. The infusion rate should be adjusted per hour to ensure that serum glucose falls by at least 50 mg/dL/h. The insulin infusion rate may be decreased by 0.05 U/kg per hour until a rate of 0.5 U/h (minimum rate) is reached. Dextrose should be added to the intravenous fluids when the plasma glucose concentration reaches <200 mg/dL in patients with DKA and <300 mg/dL in patients with HSS. The insulin infusion should be continued to maintain a plasma glucose level of 150–200 mg/dL until ketoacidosis has resolved, as evidenced by normalization of pH and anion gap among those with DKA, and until mental status and the hyperosmolar state are corrected in HHS cases.

The use of insulin lispro or aspart in subcutaneous boluses seems to be as effective as IV regular insulin infusion and a safe alternative for patients in situations where insulin infusion is not practical. An initial bolus of 0.2–0.3 U/kg of rapid-acting insulin followed by maintenance boluses of 0.1–0.2 U/kg every hour to 2 h may be used. Once glucose is less than 250, consider reducing the maintenance boluses until resolution of the DKA.

Electrolytes

Potassium Therapy   The initial insulin-deficit state, hypertonicity, and acidosis lead to a shift of potassium from the intracellular to the extracellular compartment in the setting of total body

potassium deficit of 3–5 mmol/kg. Fluid and insulin therapy promote a rapid intracellular shift of potassium, which may result in
hypokalemia with the risk of arrhythmia and even cardiac arrest.
Hence, early IV potassium therapy should be initiated when the
serum potassium level is below 5.0 mEq/L with the goal of maintaining a potassium level of 4–5 mEq/L during therapy. An exception to this rule is the case of low urine output or severely decreased
renal function whereby potassium should be given only if low and
monitored carefully.

Bicarbonate Therapy   The use of bicarbonate in DKA is controversial. The current ADA guidelines recommend bicarbonate
therapy for the severe metabolic acidosis with a serum pH <6.9.
However, no study has shown benefit from the use of this therapy.
Bicarbonate use has some potential side effects including cerebral
edema, hypokalemia, rebound acidosis, hypoxia, and hypernatremia. In view of the lack of evidence of a therapeutic effect, it
should generally be avoided.

Phosphate Therapy   Replace if serum phosphate is less than
1 mg/dL, especially in a patient with evidence of respiratory or
cardiac distress. If the phosphate level is higher than 1 mg/dL, it
usually will self-correct once the patient has resumed eating.
There is no evidence of a beneficial effect of phosphate replacement, and aggressive intravenous phosphate therapy can cause
hypocalcemia; therefore, in case of phosphate replacement, calcium levels should be monitored closely.

Monitoring

All patients should get frequent clinical and laboratory reas-
sessment to ensure an adequate glycemic control, adequate
urine output, and electrolyte correction and avoid fluid overload. The main assessments include finger-stick blood glucose
(every hour to prevent hypoglycemia) and at least basic metabolic panel (every 1–4 hours to monitor potassium levels and
the anion gap).

Criteria for Resolution

Criteria for establishing the resolution of DKA include a serum glucose ≤250 mg/dL and at least two of the following criteria: normalization of the anion gap, a venous or arterial pH ≥7.3, and a serum bicarbonate level ≥18 mEq/L. Ketonemia and ketonuria may persist for 24–36 h due to delayed ketone elimination. Patients who recover from ketoacidosis may develop a secondary hyperchloremic non-anion gap metabolic acidosis resulting from aggressive saline administration. The serum bicarbonate may not normalize immediately for this reason as it is temporarily "replaced" by chloride. In HHS, resolution may be declared when a plasma glucose level ≤250 mg/dL and normal effective serum osmolarity <310 mOsmol/kg are achieved in the setting of a restored baseline mental status.

Complications

Hypoglycemia: 5–25% of the patients with DKA develop hypoglycemia. This is due to a significant percentage of patients presenting with hyperglycemic emergencies have a defective adrenergic response to low blood sugar. Therefore, a lack of frequent monitoring, not adjusting the insulin dose appropriately and not adding dextrose-containing solutions when blood sugar is less than 200 mg/dL, can easily lead to hypoglycemia.

Hypokalemia can occur when insulin therapy is started with serum potassium less than 3.3 mEq/L because of the mechanisms discussed in electrolyte management section.

Cerebral edema is rare in adults. However, the mortality in children, where it is seen more often, can be as high as 20–40%. Fluctuation in the mental status, abnormal verbal or motor response to pain, decorticate or decerebrate posturing, cranial nerve palsy, and abnormal neurogenic respiratory pattern have been described. Onset is usually 4–12 h after starting treatment of DKA. The mechanism of cerebral edema is not well understood. Either mannitol 0.5–1 g/kg IV over 20 min or 3% saline fluid 5–10 ml/kg can be used. After initiating treatment, monitoring for thrombosis, cerebral infraction and hemorrhage is indicated.

Rhabdomyolysis, more common in HHS than DKA, can lead to renal failure. Checking creatine kinase every 2–3 h in patients with myalgia, weakness, and dark urine is recommended.

Transition of Care

Transition to a subcutaneous insulin regimen is indicated when the acute metabolic derangement has resolved and the patient is alert and can start oral nutrition. For patients who remain critically ill (e.g., shock requiring pressor agents, mechanical ventilation) or will undergo additional interventions (e.g., surgery), insulin infusion therapy should be continued. The half-life of intravenous regular human insulin is less than 10 min. Therefore, when transitioning from IV insulin to subcutaneous insulin, abrupt interruptions of the insulin infusion should be avoided. An overlap for 2–4 h of the insulin infusion and subcutaneous basal insulin is absolutely necessary to avoid rebound hyperglycemia and possible reopening of the anion gap from ketoacidosis.

To choose a subcutaneous insulin regimen for a patient with controlled diabetes, home insulin regimen can be restarted if appropriate. However, for patients with uncontrolled diabetes and insulin-naïve or newly diagnosed diabetes, insulin can be started at a total daily dose of 0.5–0.8 U/kg/dL, 50% administered as long-acting basal insulin and the other 50% in pre-meal boluses of rapid-acting insulin analogs trying to mimic normal insulin physiology. Long-acting insulin analogs seem to have a lower incidence of hypoglycemia compared to intermediate-acting insulin (neutral protamine Hagedorn, NPH). Evidence suggests that administration of insulin glargine at a dose of 0.25 U/kg within 12 h of initiation of intravenous insulin infusion may help prevent rebound hyperglycemia following acute management of DKA. Chronic hyperglycemia leads to structural and functional damage in the beta cells decreasing the secretion of insulin and also interferes with the action of insulin in the target tissue causing insulin resistance. Therefore once hyperglycemia improves, insulin sensitivity changes quickly, and insulin dose adjustment may be required after recovery from acute illness, especially in those with renal or pancreatic insufficiency.

Disposition

With proper treatment, the average time to the resolution of anion gap acidosis is 3 h. If the hyperglycemic crisis itself resolves in the emergency department, these patients may be stable enough for general floor admission to continue subcutaneous insulin, pending improved volume status after resuscitation, closed anion gap, and ability to tolerate fluids by the mouth. Patients with severe DKA or HHS often require ICU admission for adequate treatment, observation, and resolution of sepsis, hypoxia, altered mental status, hypotension, persistent tachycardia, severe acidosis, or electrolyte abnormalities. Acute comorbidities such as myocardial infarction or cerebrovascular accidents may also dictate disposition to an ICU. If the patient has to stay in the emergency department longer than expected, the patient can be managed in the proper-staffed observation unit, and the need of ICU admission can be obviated.

It is important to evaluate the cause of acute hyperglycemic emergency and treat it to prevent recurrence. DKA is the initial presentation of diabetes in approximately 15–20% of adults and 30–40% of children with type 1 diabetes. Early identification of new-onset diabetes in the emergency department can prompt the timely inclusion of a multidisciplinary team including an endocrinologist, dietitian, and social worker with ability to provide diabetes education and arrange outpatient follow-up appointment that can prevent future hospital admissions.

Visual impairment can lead to inappropriate dosing of insulin specially when using vials of insulin preparation; in these cases, an insulin pen should be considered. For patients with severe visual impairment and, also, for patients with cognitive impairment, supervised or assisted insulin injection should be arranged with home health care, family members, or assisted living facilities/nursing home admission to prevent readmission with hyperglycemic crisis.

Lipodystrophy due to repetitive insulin injection in the same area and malnourished patients with low fat mass should be counseled about the appropriate technique and area to inject insulin.

In patients presenting to the emergency department with hyperglycemic emergencies due to medication nonadherence, especially in those with multiple recent readmissions, further questioning should aim to identify the reason behind the medication noncompliance, which in most cases is due to socioeconomic issues.

In about half of the patients presenting with DKA or HHS due to medication nonadherence, the underlying problem is an inability to afford medication. In the United States, insulin can be very expensive and almost unaffordable for patients without insurance. For these patients, early social worker involvement may help the patient find community resources for insulin availability. For patients with limited access to health care, for example, undocumented patients, the physician should be aware of inexpensive options in the community such as state programs, health department free options, and local pharmacies where they can purchase insulin without prescriptions.

When prescribing insulin, even patients with insurance can have difficulties obtaining the insulin brand prescribed. Depending on the insurance, prescribing the right brand of insulin with the lowest copayment for the patient can make a big difference in compliance and, therefore, can prevent the next episode of DKA or HHS (Table 25.1).

Table 25.1 Differences between DKA and HHS

DKA	HHS
Severe insulin deficiency with excess of counterregulatory hormones, promoting gluconeogenesis, glycogenolysis, and ketone formation	Relative insulin deficiency and inadequate fluid intake, leading to gluconeogenesis and glycogenolysis
Glucose levels usually 300–500 mg/dL	>600 mg/dL
Plasma osmolarity <320	>320
Ketones in blood and urine	Absent
Metabolic acidosis with anion gap	Normal pH
Elevated beta-hydroxybutyrate	Absent
Most common symptoms: abdominal pain, nausea, vomiting	Most common symptoms: polyuria, polydipsia, and altered mental status
Acute onset	Subacute onset

Suggested Reading

American Diabetes Association. Summary of revisions: standards of medical care in diabetes—2018. Diabetes Care. 2018;41(Suppl 1):S4–6. https://doi.org/10.2337/dc18-Srev01.

CDC. New CDC report: More than 100 million Americans have diabetes or prediabetes. July 18, 2017. Available online https://www.cdc.gov/media/releases/2017/p0718-diabetes-report.html.

Crilly CJ, Allen AJ, Amato TM, Tiberio A, Schulman RC, Silverman RA. Evaluating the Emergency Department Observation Unit for the management of hyperglycemia in adults. Am J Emerg Med. 2018;36(11):1975–9. https://doi.org/10.1016/j.ajem.2018.02.027. Epub 2018 Feb 27.

Echouffo-Tcheugui JB, Garg R. Management of hyperglycemia and diabetes in the Emergency Department. Curr Diab Rep. 2017;17(8):56. https://doi.org/10.1007/s11892-017-0883-2.

Fayfman M, Pasquel FJ, Umpierrez GE. Management of hyperglycemic crises: diabetic ketoacidosis and hyperglycemic hyperosmolar state. Med Clin North Am. 2017;101(3):587–606. https://doi.org/10.1016/j.mcna.2016.12.011.

Management of Preexisting Diabetes and Gestational Diabetes During Hospitalization

Gregory P. Westcott
and Florence M. Brown

Contents

G. P. Westcott
Beth Israel Deaconess Medical Center and Joslin Diabetes Center,
Department of Endocrinology, Diabetes and Metabolism, Boston, MA,
USA
e-mail: gregory.westcott@joslin.harvard.edu

F. M. Brown (✉)
Joslin-Beth Israel Deaconess Medical Center Diabetes in Pregnancy
Program, Joslin Diabetes Center, Department of Adult Diabetes, Boston,
MA, USA
e-mail: florence.brown@joslin.harvard.edu

© Springer Nature Switzerland AG 2020
R. K. Garg et al. (eds.), *Handbook of Inpatient Endocrinology*,
https://doi.org/10.1007/978-3-030-38976-5_26

Differentiate Between Preexisting Diabetes and Gestational Diabetes

When evaluating patients hospitalized during pregnancy, it is important to determine whether they have preexisting type 1 or type 2 diabetes, or whether they have gestational diabetes. Knowing their preconception diagnosis and treatment as well as the circumstances of their diagnosis provides insights into their current treatment and eventual postpartum care.

Definition of Gestational Diabetes (See Table 26.1)

As opposed to preexisting diabetes, gestational diabetes mellitus (GDM) is diagnosed during pregnancy. GDM screening is typically performed at 24–28 weeks of gestation when insulin

Table 26.1 ADA diagnostic criteria for gestational diabetes

Diagnosis of gestational diabetes		Glucose in mg/dl
One-step method	75 g	Fasting: ≥92, 1 h: ≥180, 2 h: ≥153 One abnormal value required
Two-step method	Step 1: 50 g Step 2: 100 g	Non-fasting: 1 h: ≥130 to ≥140 (institutional) Fasting: ≥95, 1 h: ≥180, 2 h: ≥155, 3 h: ≥140, usually two abnormal values required

resistance has increased and hyperglycemia is usually apparent upon testing. Diagnosing GDM has been controversial. Recommendations have shifted over time and differ by organization. The 2018 American Diabetes Association (ADA) guidelines propose two diagnostic protocol options: a one-step fasting 75 g oral glucose tolerance test (OGTT) and a two-step evaluation which includes a 50 g non-fasting screen followed by a fasting 100 g OGTT for those who screen positive. The one-step OGTT employs glucose cutoffs of $\geq$92 mg/dL fasting, $\geq$180 mg/dL at 1 h, and/or $\geq$153 mg/dL at 2 h with one abnormal value indicating a positive test. The non-fasting 50 g screen, also called a glucose loading test (GLT), uses cutoffs which range from $\geq$130 mg/dL to $\geq$140 mg/dL at 1 h, depending on institutional guidelines. The subsequent fasting 100 g OGTT is positive when at least two (or one, depending on the guideline used) of the following cutoffs, proposed by Carpenter and Coustan, are met: $\geq$95 mg/dL fasting, $\geq$180 mg/dL at 1 h, $\geq$155 mg/dL at 2 h, or $\geq$140 mg/dL at 3 h. The Carpenter-Coustan cutoffs have been demonstrated to confer additional benefit with respect to pregnancy-induced hypertension, shoulder dystocia, cesarean delivery, and macrosomia compared to the less stringent criteria from the National Diabetes Data Group, which uses OGTT cutoffs 5–10 mg/dL higher than Carpenter-Coustan. The one-step method is a more sensitive method to detect gestational hyperglycemia, and data from the Hyperglycemia and Adverse Pregnancy Outcome (HAPO) trial suggested that there is a continuous relationship between maternal glucose and primary cesarean section delivery, neonatal hypoglycemia, birth weight over the 90th percentile, and cord C-peptide over the 90th percentile, and the one-step method is therefore the method endorsed by the International Association of Diabetes and Pregnancy Study Groups (IADPSG). The complexities of the debate between the one-step and two-step methods include discussions of changes in prevalence of diagnosis, effects of outcomes, and medical costs.

Women at high risk of abnormal glucose metabolism should be evaluated during the first trimester. The 2018 ACOG Practice Bulletin expanded list of criteria for patients considered high risk are those with:

- High-risk race or ethnicity
- Hypertension
- HDL cholesterol less than 35 mg/dL or triglyceride level over 250 mg/dL
- Polycystic ovarian syndrome or clinical conditions associated with insulin resistance such as acanthosis nigricans
- History of cardiovascular disease
- Obesity
- GDM during a previous pregnancy
- Previous baby with birth weight over 9 pounds
- Glycosuria
- Having a first-degree relative with diabetes
- Impaired fasting glucose

These women should be evaluated with the one-step fasting 75 g 2 h OGTT. A screening GLT is not indicated in this high-risk population, as the sensitivity of this test is approximately 80% and therefore may be negative in 20% of patients with GDM.

Note that alternative measures may also be incorporated in determining fetal and maternal risk. An A1c value ≥ 5.9 during the first trimester is associated with congenital malformations, pre-eclampsia, shoulder dystocia, and perinatal death. Note that while an A1c ≤ 5.9 has a high negative predictive value for ruling out overt diabetes, it is not highly sensitive in diagnosing gestational diabetes. Therefore, screening should be reassessed at 24–28 weeks of gestation with either the one-step or the two-step method for women with A1c <5.9% on early screening.

Glycemic Targets (See Table 26.2)

Glycemic targets are the same regardless of whether the patient has preexisting or gestational diabetes. ADA and the American College of Obstetricians and Gynecologists (ACOG) accepted targets are <95 mg/dL fasting and postprandial targets of <140 mg/dL at 1 h and <120 mg/dL at 2 h after a meal commences (typically patients measure either 1 or 2 h postprandial blood glucose, not both). However, it is noteworthy that in the normal pregnant populations, mean ± SD for fasting blood glucose is 71 mg ± 8 mg/

Table 26.2 Glycemic targets for pregnant women with diabetes

Glycemic targets	Glucose in mg/dl
Antepartum *ACOG and ADA 2018* *Joslin* *Fetal AC ≥75th percentile (GDM only)*	Fasting: <95, 1 h PP: <140, 2 h PP: <120 Fasting: <95[a] or <99[b], 1 h PP: <130 Fasting: 60–79, 1 h PP: 90–109
Labor and delivery	80–110
Postpartum	Fasting: <100, 2 h PP: <140

PP postprandial
[a]GDM
[b]Preexisting DM

dl, and post-meal blood glucose at 1 h is 109+/−13 mg/dl and at 2 h is 99.3 ± 10 mg/dl, which are considerably lower than the upper ranges of these targets. So, some institutions advocate lowering the upper range of targets; for example, Joslin Diabetes Center recommends 1 h postprandial glucose target of 100–129 mg/dl. For patients with gestational diabetes, more stringent glycemic targets should be considered in patients with a fetus whose Hadlock abdominal circumference (AC) is ≥75th percentile prior to 34 weeks of gestation. The fetal AC discriminates low and high risk for large-for-gestational-age newborns. When high-risk fetal AC growth is identified, lower glucose targets significantly reduce excessive fetal growth. Therefore, fasting glucose target of 60–79 mg/dL and 1 h postprandial target of 90–109 mg/dL are recommended in these patients. Note that this guidance applies specifically to gestational diabetes, since there is no evidence to support similar adjustments in preexisting type 1 or 2 diabetes. In women with preexisting diabetes, these targets may be quite difficult to achieve without increasing the risk of significant hypoglycemia.

Treatment Options

There is considerable overlap between outpatient and inpatient management of diabetes during pregnancy. In addition to monitoring blood glucose while fasting and at peak post meal, patients diagnosed with gestational diabetes and preexisting diabetes are advised to adhere to consistent carbohydrate intake with small frequent meals, for example: 30 g of carbohydrates for breakfast and 45 g for lunch and dinner with 15–20 g snacks between meals and before bed. Fasting urine ketone measurement in the morning helps identify patients who are over-restricting carbohydrates. Counseling should be provided on the quality of the diet. To conceptualize a healthy diet, we recommend the "Healthy Plate" in which half the plate is filled with non-starchy vegetables, one-quarter with whole grains, and one-quarter with lean protein. Fats are derived primarily from plant sources. Low-impact exercise is also encouraged.

Patients with Gestational Diabetes

Patients with gestational diabetes who maintain blood glucose within target ranges with lifestyle interventions alone are classified as having GDMA1. For patients who are unable to maintain glucose within target range without over-restricting carbohydrates, insulin is recommended. If there is no history of preexisting diabetes, patients who require insulin to maintain target glucose concentrations are classified as having GDMA2. In gestational diabetes, the pattern of hyperglycemia should guide the choice of insulin. To reduce fasting hyperglycemia, NPH at bedtime is considered standard of care. Insulin analogues aspart and lispro can be dosed before the meal to manage postprandial hyperglycemia, typically via a fixed premeal dose that can be titrated to achieve glycemic target. As mealtime insulin doses are up-titrated to control postprandial glucose peak, hypoglycemia prior to the subsequent meal is common and should be prevented with a small snack 2–3 h after the meal.

The use of oral medications during pregnancy has been controversial. Until recently, ACOG had endorsed the use of glyburide and metformin for gestational diabetes despite the fact that the FDA has not approved the medications for this indication, while the ADA has stated that insulin is the first-line therapy for

GDM and type 2 diabetes in pregnancy. ACOG has now also embraced this view and considers insulin the preferred treatment for diabetes during pregnancy. Because glyburide crosses the placenta, it can contribute to fetal hyperinsulinemia, and there is evidence that it increases the risk of macrosomia, preeclampsia, neonatal hypoglycemia, and hyperbilirubinemia. Metformin crosses the placenta, has high failure rates, and achieves therapeutic levels in the fetus, and recently published data from the metformin in gestational diabetes trial found that at 9 years, offspring of women who received metformin during pregnancy were larger by weight, arm and waist circumference, waist-to-height ratio, BMI, triceps skinfold, and MRI abdominal fat volume.

Patients with Type 1 Diabetes

Patients with type 1 diabetes typically continue their current regimen with either multiple-dose injections or insulin pump therapy. This includes basal insulin and mealtime insulin administered as fixed doses or determined by a ratio of insulin to calculated carbohydrate intake in combination with correctional insulin based on a correction factor or sliding scale. Insulin detemir is non-inferior to NPH insulin for basal dosing based on results from a randomized controlled trial. Glargine is not recommended in pregnant patients or in those planning a pregnancy, as there is no randomized controlled trial outcome data comparing it to detemir or NPH insulin. There is a six- to eightfold increased affinity of glargine for the IGF-1 receptor, which is of hypothetical concern, although insulin does not cross the placenta and therefore is unlikely to contribute to increased fetal growth. Insulin analogues aspart and lispro are preferred for mealtime dosing as above. Glulisine and degludec have not been studied in pregnancy. Insulin requirements vary throughout pregnancy in all patients on insulin, increasing in the first 9 weeks of gestation, decreasing in weeks 9–16, increasing again until week 37, and then decreasing again in the final month until delivery. Patients with type 1 diabetes may also benefit from continuous glucose monitoring.

Patients with Type 2 Diabetes

Patients with type 2 diabetes should be treated exclusively with insulin. There is inadequate safety data regarding the use of GLP-1 agonists, DPP-4 inhibitors, alpha glucosidase inhibitors, and SGLT2 inhibitors in pregnancy.

Diabetic Retinopathy

In women with preexisting type 1 or type 2 diabetes, a dilated eye exam should be performed in each trimester of pregnancy with the frequency of follow-up depending on the level of baseline retinopathy. The level of retinopathy and the timing of the last dilated eye exam should be determined in all hospitalized patients. For patients who require prolonged hospitalization, an ophthalmology consultation may be necessary.

Special Situations

Diabetic Ketoacidosis

DKA may occur at lower glucose levels than what is typically seen in the nongravid state (<200 mg/dl) due to the flux of glucose from the maternal to the fetal circulation via glucose transporter-1 (GLUT-1), the lowered renal threshold for glucose leading to enhanced glycosuria due to reduced tubular reabsorption capacity and increased GFR, and the accelerated starvation state that contributes to ketonemia. Infection, insulin omission or failed delivery, or the use of medications such as terbutaline or glucocorticoids may predispose to DKA. When a patient is seen in triage or as an inpatient due to concern for DKA, insulin pump infusion issues should be ruled-out and insulin given by syringe or intravenously if needed, adequate hydration ensured, and electrolyte abnormalities corrected. Insulin drip protocols should be employed when necessary. Intravenous dextrose may be required to maintain mild hyperglycemia (150–200 mg/dl) to allow for adequate insulin infusion until the anion gap is closed and the bicarbonate level has normalized. In a recent study, fetal demise occurred in 15.6% of DKA in pregnancy cases; the need for maternal ICU admission and higher serum osmolality were risk factors for fetal demise.

Betamethasone Therapy

Betamethasone is often given in the setting of preterm labor as it has been shown to reduce perinatal mortality and incidence of respiratory distress syndrome in infants delivered before 34 weeks. It is typically given in two doses of 12 mg 24 h apart. An algorithm developed by Mathiesen and others helps proactively adjust insulin dosing to prevent severe glycemic abnormalities. On the day of the first betamethasone dose, the evening insulin dose should be increased by 25%. All insulin doses should be increased (compared to baseline dose) by 45% on day 2, by 40% on day 3, by 30% on day 4, and by 10% on day 5. On days 6 and 7, insulin doses may be reduced toward original dosing, with the caveat that requirements may not return completely to pre-glucocorticoid dosing, as baseline insulin resistance has likely increased as the pregnancy has advanced.

Labor and Delivery

Glycemic Targets

Careful monitoring of blood glucose during labor and delivery is required. Since intrapartum glucose levels affect the risk of neonatal hypoglycemia, the risk is lowest when maternal intrapartum glucose levels average <100 mg/dL while aiming for a range between 80 and 110 mg/dL.

Treatment Strategies

In the setting of planned induction of labor or preeclampsia requiring magnesium infusion, oral intake may be decreased or eliminated for several hours. For patients with GDM or type 2 diabetes, basal insulin doses may need to be reduced or held, depending on the timing of expected delivery, and prandial doses likewise held or reduced based on intake status. For patients with type 1 diabetes, an intravenous insulin drip is preferred while the patient is NPO during labor, delivery, and immediately postdelivery. An ideal insulin drip protocol will include insulin and dextrose infusions that can be titrated hourly by nursing staff based on finger-stick blood glucose data. When oral intake is resumed, the transition back to subcutaneous insulin can be accomplished by overlapping basal (2 h) and prandial insulin (1 h) with the insulin drip. An insulin drip can also be used in patients with GDM or type 2 diabetes if intrapartum blood glucose is difficult to control.

Postpartum

Postdelivery Insulin Requirements

Following delivery, there is a significant decrease in insulin resistance as placental hormones clear. Patients with GDM typically do not require insulin following delivery, and it should be discontinued. Patients with type 2 diabetes who were not on insulin prior to conception may also be trialed off insulin. Oral medications should be held as long as the patient is breastfeeding since these medications distribute to breast milk. Postpartum blood glucose can be monitored following delivery to confirm a return to normal levels (<100 mg/dL fasting and <140 mg/dL at 2 h postprandially). Patients with type 1 diabetes typically require a reduction of insulin doses to approximately 50% of preconception dose. Breastfeeding is considered beneficial due to increased insulin sensitivity and weight loss and should be encouraged for at least 6 months if possible.

After Discharge and Future Pregnancies

For patients with GDM, the postpartum period is a key opportunity for counseling regarding interventions to reduce the risk of developing type 2 diabetes in the future. The risk of developing type 2 diabetes is approximately 50% at 5–10 years after delivery. Dietary and exercise modifications should be encouraged, and if preconception BMI was ≥25 (or ≥23 for Asians), a goal of 7% weight loss compared to preconception weight will reduce the probability of developing type 2 diabetes in the future. All patients with GDM should undergo a 75 g 2 h OGTT at 6 weeks postpartum to assess for impaired glucose metabolism or type 2 diabetes. They should also be screened for GDM or undiagnosed type 2 diabetes early in subsequent pregnancies. Prior to discharge, patients with type 1 or type 2 diabetes should be advised to schedule appointments 2 weeks and 6 weeks postpartum with their outpatient endocrinologist as insulin sensitivity will be returning to baseline and insulin dosing may require adjustment. The 6 weeks postpartum visit should also include labs for A1c, creatinine, and urine albumin/creatinine ratio, and TSH should be checked given the risk of postpartum thyroiditis particularly in patients with type 1 diabetes and to monitor postpartum levothyroxine dosing changes in patients with type 1 DM who have concurrent chronic lymphocytic thyroiditis. Counseling on contraceptive options and the optimal timing of the next eye exam and endocrinology follow-up should be provided.

Suggested Reading

American Diabetes Association. 13. Management of diabetes in pregnancy: standards of medical care in diabetes—2018. Diabetes Care. 2018;41(Suppl 1):S137–S43.

Brown FM, Wyckoff J. Application of one-step IADPSG versus two-step diagnostic criteria for gestational diabetes in the real world: impact on health services, clinical care, and outcomes. Curr Diab Rep. 2017;17(10):85.

Committee on Practice Bulletins—Obstetrics. ACOG practice bulletin no. 190: gestational diabetes mellitus. Obstet Gynecol. 2018;131(2): e49–64.

Garcia-Patterson A, Gich I, Amini SB, Catalano PM, de Leiva A, Corcoy R. Insulin requirements throughout pregnancy in women with type 1 diabetes mellitus: three changes of direction. Diabetologia. 2010;53(3):446–51.

Harvard School of Public Health. Healthy eating plate & healthy eating pyramid. 2011. https://www.hsph.harvard.edu/nutritionsource/healthy-eating-plate.

International Association of Diabetes and Pregnancy Study Groups Consensus Panel. International association of diabetes and pregnancy study groups recommendations on the diagnosis and classification of hyperglycemia in pregnancy. Diabetes Care. 2010;33(3):676–82.

Joslin Diabetes Center. Joslin diabetes center and Joslin clinic guideline for detection and management of diabetes in pregnancy. 2017. https://www.joslin.org/docs/Pregnancy-Guidelines_11-13-2016_corrected_1-11-2017.pdf.

Kjos SL, Schaefer-Graf UM. Modified therapy for gestational diabetes using high-risk and low-risk fetal abdominal circumference growth to select strict versus relaxed maternal glycemic targets. Diabetes Care. 2007;30(Suppl 2):S200–5.

Mathiesen ER, Christensen AB, Hellmuth E, Hornnes P, Stage E, Damm P. Insulin dose during glucocorticoid treatment for fetal lung maturation in diabetic pregnancy: test of an algorithm [correction of algorithm]. Acta Obstet Gynecol Scand. 2002;81(9):835–9.

The HAPO Study Cooperative Research Group. Hyperglycemia and adverse pregnancy outcomes. N Engl J Med. 2008;358(19):1991–2002.

Inpatient Insulin Pump Management

27

Maria Vamvini and Elena Toschi

Contents

M. Vamvini · E. Toschi (✉)
Adult Clinic, Joslin Diabetes Center, Harvard Medical School,
Beth Israel Deaconess Medical Center, Department of Endocrinology
and Diabetes, Boston, MA, USA
e-mail: maria.vamvini@joslin.harvard.edu;
elena.toschi@joslin.harvard.edu

© Springer Nature Switzerland AG 2020
R. K. Garg et al. (eds.), *Handbook of Inpatient Endocrinology*,
https://doi.org/10.1007/978-3-030-38976-5_27

Insulin Pump Use in the Hospital in Non-critically Ill Patients

Assess Preadmission Diabetes Status

The hospital physician should obtain a detailed medical and diabetes history including duration of diabetes, type of diabetes, presence of any complications, and review of most recent A1c. If A1c has not been checked in the past 3 months, patient should have a repeat A1c checked at the time of admission. The type of insulin pump and insulin formulation (Humalog or Novolog) as well as pump settings including basal rates, insulin-to-carbohydrate ratio/s (I:CHO), and the correction or sensitivity factor/s should be clearly documented. Pump settings also include target glucose (see Table 27.1).

Table 27.1 Insulin order for the self-administering insulin pump

Name of Insulin Pump:					
Type of Insulin:					
Target glucose:					
Settings:					
Time	Basal (U/hour)	Time	I:CHO (U/g carb)	Time	CF/SF (U/mg/dl)
MN–6 AM	0.6	MN–6 AM	1:10	MN–8 AM	1:50
6 AM–12 PM	0.8	6 AM–10 AM	1:8	8 AM–8 PM	1:35
12 PM–8 PM	0.7	10 AM–4 PM	1:10	8 PM–MN	1:50
8 PM–MN	0.5	4 PM–8 PM	1:12		
Total basal	X	8 PM–MN	1:15		

A focused physical examination assessing body weight and skin sites used for pump infusion set should be performed. The pump site should be inspected for possible pump site issues including ecchymosis, hypo- and hypertrophy, infection, and leaking. Careful assessment for diabetic neuropathy and vascular disease should be conducted.

Patients Who Can Continue Using Their Insulin Pump

Patients on insulin pump therapy are usually knowledgeable about insulin pump technology and management. These patients should be allowed to use their insulin pumps in the hospital setting if they are deemed physically, cognitively, and emotionally able to do so. Basal rates may need to be lowered (generally to about 80%) to prevent hypoglycemia. Patient and team should discuss insulin regimen changes recommended while in the hospital. Target glycemic goals may differ between staff team and patient and, therefore, both communication and documentation of recommended glucose targets are important for safe and satisfactory care. In non-critically ill hospitalized patients, both the American Diabetes Association (ADA) and Endocrine Society recommend goal for fasting and pre-meal blood glucose (BG) is <140 mg/dl and random glucose <180 mg/dl.

For contraindications for insulin pump use, see section "Contraindications for Self-Administered Insulin Pump Therapy".

Assess Current Nutritional Status

All patients with diabetes should follow a consistent carbohydrate meal plan while in the hospital. Many hospitalized patients are rendered nothing per oral (NPO) for a variety of reasons (impending surgery or diagnostic procedures, gastrointestinal disease, inability to eat). It is important that the reason and anticipated duration of NPO status are documented. Any special dietary restrictions should be noted. If a patient is getting enteral tube feedings, note the content, rate, and times of tube feeds. Similar data need to be collected for parenteral nutrition. Based on this information, insulin pump settings may need to be adjusted. In patients who are NPO, it is recommended that the basal rate should be decreased by 20–50%. In cyclical enteral tube feeding, basal rates may need to be increased 2 hours prior to initiation of the feeding cycle, initially by 20%, and then titrated upward as needed. In patients receiving total parenteral nutrition (TPN), basal rate may need to be adjusted depending on the amount of carbohydrates (dextrose) in each TPN bag.

Assess Other Medications That May Affect Glycemic Status

Most hospitalized patients are likely to be receiving one or more medications that can potentially affect their blood glucose levels. Most commonly used medications are the glucocorticoids. Basal rates as well as insulin-to-carb ratio and sensitivity factor should be adjusted to mitigate glucocorticoid-induced hyperglycemia.

If possible, medications for intravenous (IV) infusion should be prepared in glucose-free solutions rather than in dextrose in water.

Medical Orders for Insulin Pump Treatment

In order to allow a given patient to continue using an insulin pump, a medication order for the insulin pump must be provided by a licensed independent practitioner. A medication order to allow a patient to continue using an insulin pump includes acknowledgment that the patient has been assessed to be competent in operating the pump and that no exclusion criteria apply (see section "Contraindications for Self-Administered Insulin Pump Therapy"). The orders for the self-administering insulin pump should include type of insulin, basal rate, and bolus doses for meals (insulin-to-carb ratio) and for hyperglycemia correction (insulin sensitivity or correction factor) along with glucose targets (Table 27.1). The order should also dictate the frequency of blood glucose monitoring. It is optimal that an insulin pump order in the electronic medical record prompts the practitioner to obtain an endocrinology and nutrition consultation, if this is a possibility at a given institution.

Insulin Pump Management

If a medication order for insulin pump self-administration has been activated, the patient will be considered responsible for programming his/her insulin pump and changing the infusion set as per his/her own regimen (change infusion set is recommended every 2–3 days). Blood glucose should be checked at least four times a day before meals and before bedtime or every 4 hours for NPO patients. Documentation should be completed utilizing an insulin pump flowsheet (see Fig. 27.1). It is important that BG data are reviewed at least once daily by the treating team or endocrinologist for insulin dose adjustments. Basal insulin should be adjusted to keep fasting BG <140 mg/dL, and nutritional insulin should be adjusted to maintain all other BG levels in 100–180 mg/dl range. Insulin doses should be increased or decreased by 10–20% at a time to produce a meaningful effect.

The insertion site should be assessed at every shift and if glucose values >250 mg/dl. All infusion sets shall be changed by the patient at least every 72 hours. It is good practice to record the date and time of the last infusion set change once the patient is admitted to the hospital.

Indications to change infusion sets more frequently may include but are not limited to:

- The site is erythematous, swollen, or warm to touch.
- Bleeding at insertion site.
- Discomfort at insertion site.
- Unresolved delivery alarm alerts.
- The patient has two consecutive blood glucose readings greater than 250 mg/dl which are refractory to correction boluses.

	1	2	3	4	5	6AM	7	8	9	10	11	12PM
BG (mg/dL)						201						154
Carbs (g)						30						45
Meal Bolus (units)						3						4.5
Correction Bolus (units)						1						0
Basal (u/hr)						0.5						0.7

Fig. 27.1 Insulin pump flowsheet

Insulin Pump Use in the Hospital in Critically Ill Patients

It is recommended that critically ill patients not use their insulin pump. Instead they should be transitioned to intravenous insulin treatment. Intravenous insulin treatment should start as per usual in-hospital protocol. ADA recommends for most ICU patients glucose targets between 140 and 180 mg/dl.

Contraindications for Self-Administered Insulin Pump Therapy

• Acute change in conscious state/mental status as assessed by nurse or treating team
• Some procedures involving anesthesia that alter the patient's capability to manage the pump for longer period of time (>12 hours)
• Inability to demonstrate competence with pump management
• Risk of suicide or suicidal ideation
• Recurrent or persistent episodes of hypoglycemia or hyperglycemia
• Patient refusal or inability to participate in pump management
• Inability to procure their own supplies (reservoirs and infusion sets should be changed at least every 72 hours)
• Unresolved pump failure

- Unexplained hyperglycemia
- Diabetic ketoacidosis and hyperglycemic hyperosmolar state
- Unexplained, persistent hypoglycemia
- Lack of pump supplies
- Health-care decision or lack of trained health-care personnel on management of insulin pump therapy

Special Considerations Regarding Pump Therapy

Insulin Pump Use in the Hospital in Patients Undergoing Surgical Procedures

In procedures and surgeries requiring moderate sedation or anesthesia, patients have limited or no ability to operate the insulin pump independently throughout the perioperative period.

In some cases, it is appropriate to discontinue the insulin pump and provide insulin therapy via an alternative route. Among reasons to consider stopping pump use are the length of the procedure, postoperative recovery time, and use of imaging perioperatively (i.e., MRI, CT scan, radiation therapy). When use of a self-administering insulin pump is contraindicated or must be stopped, the patient may require either subcutaneous insulin via syringe or an insulin drip to maintain glycemic control for the duration of time that the pump is disconnected. Blood glucose monitoring is case dependent but may be done as frequently as 1–2 hours.

In other cases, especially when patients undergo ambulatory or short-term surgical procedures lasting a few hours ($\leq$ 2 hours), continuation of the insulin pump at a basal rate administration of insulin may be appropriate. In this scenario, basal rate should be reduced by 20–50% 2 hours pre-procedure and kept at this lower rate up to 4 hours postoperatively. Blood glucose monitoring during procedures is case dependent but may be done as frequently as 1–2 hours.

In cases where an insulin pump is to continue while the patient is sedated or under anesthesia, the following is recommended:

- An order to continue the self-administering insulin pump at the basal rate is written by the primary team if the patient is under an observation status (non-inpatient) and has no existing order in place for the pump.
- Blood glucose should be checked before the procedure/surgery, hourly during procedure/surgery and following procedure/surgery.
- IV access is confirmed.
- Documentation is completed utilizing the insulin pump flowsheet.
- Insertion site is assessed pre- and post-procedure/surgery. If the insertion site is not ideally located due to the anticipated positioning of the patient, it is recommended that the patient should move the site to a more ideal location. Infusion site and tubing should be taped to secure placement and avoid dislodging during procedure.

During Imaging Studies

During imaging or procedures utilizing x-ray, the pump should be covered by lead apron. Prior to an MRI, insulin pump and metal infusion set, if used, should be disconnected from the patient in the MRI scanning suite (a minimum of 8 feet away from MRI machine) because of incompatibility with the MRI scanning environment. Interruption of insulin infusion should be overall less than 60 min, and blood glucose levels should be monitored. If duration of the imaging study is long and the pump needs to be discontinued for longer periods of time, the patient may require either subcutaneous insulin administration or an insulin drip to maintain glycemic control and avoid ketosis for the duration of time that the pump is disconnected.

In Diabetic Ketoacidosis

Insulin pump failure can lead to diabetic ketoacidosis. Pump malfunction can be due to dislodgement of the infusion set and blockage or leakage of the tubing system, all causing an interruption of insulin delivery. In patients with diabetic ketoacidosis, the insulin pump must be discontinued, and they should be treated with continuous intravenous insulin administration as per hospital protocol. These patients may be transitioned back to the insulin pump after resolution of the diabetic ketoacidosis when clinically stable and when the acid-base disorder is corrected. The intravenous insulin should be overlapped with the pump restart by at least 2 hours to allow for adequate insulin absorption. Frequent BG monitoring is needed for several hours after the pump is restarted to ensure adequate glycemic control.

Peripartum

Many women with type 1 diabetes are treated with an insulin pump during pregnancy. It is recommended that the insulin pump be disconnected peripartum. An intravenous insulin drip is preferred while the patient is NPO during labor, delivery, and immediately post-delivery. During labor and delivery, the maternal blood glucose level should be kept between 80 and 110 mg/dl. After delivery, insulin requirement falls dramatically, and insulin rate should be decreased. For more details, see Chap. 26, "Management of Preexisting Diabetes and Gestational Diabetes During Hospitalization."

Transition from Continuous Subcutaneous Insulin Infusion (CSII) to Multiple Daily Injection (MDI) Insulin Regimen

When use of a self-administered insulin pump or CSII is contraindicated or must be stopped, the patient will require either subcutaneous insulin via syringe or an insulin drip to maintain glycemic control for the duration of time that the pump is disconnected. When there is no indication for treatment with an insulin drip, insulin should be administered subcutaneously through MDI. Because of varying absorption rates, subcutaneous insulin ideally needs to be initiated before discontinuation of the pump. Long-acting (basal) insulin should be administered at least 2 hours and rapid-acting insulin 30 minutes before disconnecting the pump. To transition to MDI insulin regimen, the basal dose should be calculated using the 24 hour basal dose of insulin delivered from the pump. The total basal daily insulin can be given as once-daily or twice-daily injections. Prandial insulin can be calculated as half of a patient's usual total daily dose of insulin divided by three. Alternatively, the patient, if able, should be allowed to calculate the prandial insulin using his/her insulin-to-carbohydrate ratio from the pump setting. His/her correctional insulin bolus should be calculated according to the insulin pump correction factor. Capillary blood glucose should be measured before meals and bedtime or every 4 hours if the patient is NPO.

Use of Continuous Glucose Monitor (CGM) in the Hospital

In Non-ICU Patients

There are currently no guidelines for use of CGM in the inpatient setting. Some sensors need to be calibrated, and some of them are affected from commonly used drugs such as acetaminophen. There is also a lack of evidence on accuracy during hypoxemia, hypotension, or hypothermia. Therefore, sensor readings or trends may not be accurate in the hospital setting. Thus far, the use of this technology in hospital has been largely experimental.

In ICU Patients

Two CGM systems are FDA-approved for use in hospitals: GlucoScout® (International Biomedical) and OptiScanner 5000®. However, use of CGM in critically ill patients in the ICU is not currently recommended. Data from several ICU studies have been conflicting, and there is no clear evidence that use of subcutaneous CGM systems improves the glycemic control of critically ill patients in a clinically significant manner. More large-scale studies are needed to determine potential beneficial effects from CGM use in the ICU.

Sensor-Augmented Insulin Pump and Hybrid Closed-Loop System

Sensor-augmented insulin pump and hybrid closed-loop systems which feature CGM are now available. Sensor-augmented insulin pumps can suspend insulin delivery based on CGM sensor reading to prevent hypoglycemia. Hybrid closed-loop systems not only can suspend infusion temporarily to prevent episodes of hypoglycemia but can also adjust basal insulin delivery based on sensor reading. However, patients are still required to bolus prior to meals and administer correction boluses as needed to keep these systems operating correctly. Therefore, similar criteria should be used to evaluate if the patient can operate these pumps while in hospital. The sensor-augmented insulin pump and hybrid closed-loop systems should not be used in the ICU settings.

Evaluate Diabetes Treatment at Time of Discharge

Clinical conditions may change during hospitalization necessitating changes to pre-admission treatment for diabetes. Additionally, changes to diabetes treatment may be indicated due to poor pre-admission diabetes control.

If there is a plan to discharge the patient to a rehabilitation or skilled nursing facility, case management should determine the competence of the facility to manage an insulin pump. Prior to patient transfer, the facility will be required to provide their protocol for managing patients on insulin pumps. Discharge paperwork should include the insulin pump treatment plan and a contingency plan for insulin management in case the patient is not be able to continue insulin pump therapy.

If pump use is not recommended for any reason prior to discharge, then a multiple daily injection regimen with long-acting and short-acting insulin for meals and correction doses should be provided.

Reasons to be discharged on MDI include patient preference, mental status changes precluding restarting CSII, and lack of additional supplies.

Follow-Up After Discharge

Discharge plans should include a timely follow-up visit for continued outpatient diabetes care. An appointment should be made for the patient to see their diabetes care providers within 2–4 weeks of discharge. Because glycemic control is expected to change after discharge, make sure that the patient is able to contact a diabetes care provider in case of high or low blood glucose levels.

Suggested Readings

American Diabetes Association. Diabetes care in the hospital. Diabetes Care. 2017;40(Suppl. 1):S120–7.

Garg R, Hudson M, editors. Hyperglycemia in the hospital setting. New Delhi: JP Brothers; 2014.

Grunberger G, Abelseth J, Bailey T, Bode B, Handelsman Y, Hellman R, et al. Consensus Statement by the American Association of Clinical Endocrinologists/American College of Endocrinology Insulin Pump Management Task Force. Endocr Pract. 2014;20(5).

Joslin Clinical Guidelines at https://www.joslin.org/info/joslin-clinical-guidelines.html.

Kannan S, Satra A, Calogeras E, Lock P, Lansang MC. Insulin pump patient characteristics and glucose control in the hospitalized setting. J Diabetes Sci Technol. 2014;8(3):473–8.

Mendez CE, Umpierrez GE. Management of type 1 diabetes in the hospital setting. Curr Diab Rep. 2017;17(10):98.

Peters AL, Ahmann AJ, Battelino T, Evert A, Hirschn IB, Murad MH, et al. Diabetes technology—continuous subcutaneous insulin infusion therapy and continuous glucose monitoring in adults: an endocrine society clinical practice guideline. J Clin Endocrinol Metab. 2016;101(11):3922–37.

Thompson B, Korytkowski M, Klonoff DC, Cook CB. Consensus statement on use of continuous subcutaneous insulin infusion therapy in the hospital. J Diabetes Sci Technol. 2018;12(4):880–9.

Umpierrez GE, Hellman R, Korytkowski MT, Kosiborod M, Maynard GA, Montori VM, et al. Endocrine society. management of hyperglycemia in hospitalized patients in non-critical care setting: an endocrine society clinical practice guideline. J Clin Endocrinol Metab. 2012;97(1):16–38.

Umpierrez GE, Klonoff DC. Diabetes technology update: use of insulin pumps and continuous glucose monitoring in the hospital. Diabetes Care. 2018;41(8):1579–89.

Severe Hypertriglyceridemia in the Hospitalized Patient

28

Roselyn Cristelle I. Mateo and Om P. Ganda

Contents

R. C. I. Mateo
Joslin Diabetes Center, Department of Endocrinology, Beth Israel
Deaconess Medical Center, Boston, MA, USA
e-mail: roselyn.mateo@joslin.harvard.edu

O. P. Ganda (✉)
Joslin Diabetes Center, Department of Medicine, Beth Israel
Deaconess Medical Center, Boston, MA, USA
e-mail: om.ganda@joslin.harvard.edu

© Springer Nature Switzerland AG 2020
R. K. Garg et al. (eds.), *Handbook of Inpatient Endocrinology*,
https://doi.org/10.1007/978-3-030-38976-5_28

Define Hypertriglyceridemia (HTG)

Clinical Practice Guidelines (CPG) from major professional societies, including the National Cholesterol Education Program Expert Panel on Detection, Evaluation, and Treatment of High Blood Cholesterol in Adults (NCEP ATP III), National Lipid Association (NLA), American Association of Clinical Endocrinologists (AACE), and the Endocrine Society (TES), have proposed different criteria for the clinical diagnosis of elevated triglyceride levels under fasting conditions, as shown in Table 28.1.

Severe HTG, usually >1000 mg/dl, accounts for 10–15% of cases of AP and often occurs in the setting of acute or chronic insulin deficiency. In most cases, AP requires emergency hospitalization and can be fatal, if not treated promptly, due to severe

Table 28.1 Criteria for high fasting TG

	NCEP ATP III	NLA	AACE	TES	
Normal	<150 mg/dL	<150	<150	*Normal*	<150 mg/dL
Borderline high	150–199	150–199	150–199	*Mild*	150–199
High	200–499	200–499	200–499	*Moderate*	200–999
Very high	>= 500	>= 500	>= 500	*Severe*	1000–1999
				Very severe	>= 2000

hemodynamic changes, hypovolemia, and hypotension. AP due to HTG may follow more severe clinical course than that due to other causes.

Risk Factors That Contribute to Elevated TG Levels

Severe HTG levels are usually associated with genetic traits that are often combined with acquired risk factors such as overweight, physical inactivity, insulin resistance, metabolic syndrome, advanced chronic kidney disease (CKD), or uncontrolled diabetes mellitus (DM). The underlying genetic disorders include familial hypertriglyceridemia, familial dysbetalipoproteinemia, monogenic or polygenic chylomicronemia syndrome (FCS), acquired partial lipodystrophy, and familial combined hyperlipidemia (FCH). Pregnancy, hypothyroidism, autoimmune disorders such as paraproteinemia or systemic lupus erythematosus, and certain drugs are also contributing factors to HTG (Table 28.2).

Table 28.2   Medications that may affect TG levels

Drugs	Mechanism of action
Thiazide, furosemide	Modulate adipocyte differentiation leading to accumulation of plasma TGs in susceptible patients with certain genetic polymorphisms
Beta blockers (particularly atenolol, metoprolol, and propranolol)	Peripheral vasoconstriction through peripheral β-adrenergic receptors can increase insulin resistance, leading to lowering of HDL-C, and increased TG; induce decreased TG hydrolysis through a reduction in the muscle lipoprotein lipase (LPL) and endothelial dysfunction from peripheral vasoconstriction
Estrogen	Increase the hepatic secretion of VLDL

(continued)

Table 28.2 (continued)

Drugs	Mechanism of action
Bile acid sequestrants (BAS) (cholestyramine, colestipol, colesevelam)	Activation of phosphatidic acid phosphatase promotes hepatic TG synthesis and induces secretion of TG-rich VLDL. BAS also act as farnesoid X receptor (FXR) antagonists and activate liver X receptor (LXR), thus increasing TG levels
Protease inhibitors, e.g., ritonavir and lopinavir	Increase in VLDL production and intermediate-density lipoproteins (IDL); decreased activity of lipoprotein lipase and hepatic lipase; development of insulin resistance and abnormal expression of the apolipoprotein CIII gene
Second-generation antipsychotic medications such as clozapine, olanzapine, risperidone, and quetiapine	Cause weight gain, insulin resistance, and worsening of the metabolic syndrome
Immunosuppressants (interferon, tacrolimus, sirolimus, others)	Inhibit LPL, stimulate hepatic lipogenesis
Isotretinoin	Slows down the metabolism of triglyceride-rich lipoproteins (TRL), such as chylomicrons, and remnant particles

Physical Examination

Relevant physical examination should include measurements of body mass index (BMI) and blood pressure (BP); assessment of carotid and peripheral pulses; palpation of the liver and thyroid; and inspection of palms, soles, and extensor surfaces of the arms, buttocks, trunk, and tendinous attachments. Clinical features may include eruptive xanthomas, lipemia retinalis, hepatosplenomegaly, focal neurologic symptoms such as irritability, and recurrent epigastric pain consistent with pancreatitis. Eruptive cutaneous xanthomas are filled with foam cells that appear as yellow morbilliform eruptions that measure 2–5 mm in diameter, often with erythematous areolae. Palmar crease xanthomas, typically seen in familial dyslipidemia syndrome, appear as yellow deposits within palmar creases. Lipemia retinalis is a characteristic milky appearance of the retinal vessels and pink retina. Samples of lipemic plasma develop a creamy supernatant when refrigerated overnight.

Laboratory Work-Up

Order a glucose test, thyroid function tests, and a renal panel and liver panel to detect or rule out diabetes, hypothyroidism, and renal and liver disease. Thyroid hormone plays a role in the regulation of the synthesis, metabolism, and mobilization of lipids. Patients with hypothyroidism have increased levels of total cholesterol, low-density lipoprotein cholesterol, apolipoprotein B, lipoprotein(a) levels, and triglyceride levels. Hypertriglyceridemia and reduction and dysfunction of high-density lipoprotein are also common lipid disturbances in chronic kidney disease, caused mainly by the decreased efficiency of lipoprotein lipase (LPL)-mediated very Low Density Lipoprotein-TG (VLDL-TG) lipolysis. The liver, too, plays a crucial role in the synthesis, secretion, catabolism, and storage of lipids and lipoproteins. Alcoholic and nonalcoholic liver disease affects lipid metabolism differently. High alcohol consumption can cause excessive synthesis of triglycerides, hypercholesterolemia, defective esterification of plasma cholesterol, and decreased level of high-density lipoprotein cholesterol.

Order a fasting lipid panel including total cholesterol, HDL-C, direct LDL, and TG. Hemoglobin A1c should be ordered to assess control of diabetes in the appropriate patient.

Patients with HTG may present with acute pancreatitis (AP) and relatively low amylase levels. This is brought about by interference caused by triglyceride-rich lipoprotein (TRL) that can result in falsely low amylase levels. Centrifugation before laboratory testing can remove chylomicrons from plasma and eliminate artifacts in lipemic specimens. HTG can also interfere with biochemical measurement of glucose, leading to falsely lower levels in these patients.

The Endocrine Society not only recommends against the routine measurement of lipoprotein particle heterogeneity in patients with hypertriglyceridemia but also recognizes that measurement of apolipoprotein B (Apo B) or lipoprotein(a) [Lp(a)] levels can be of value in assessing cardiovascular (CV) risk in selected cases, such as those with familial combined hyperlipidemia.

Evaluate Need for Insulin and/or Heparin Drip

HTG can contribute to adverse CV events, including acute coronary events, and AP. During AP episodes, insulin promotes synthesis and activation of lipoprotein lipase (LPL), thereby accelerating chylomicron degradation. Treatment with insulin infusion, along with hemodynamic support, can dramatically improve the hydrolysis of chylomicrons and large VLDL particles in patients with DM and uncontrolled hyperglycemia.

Heparan sulfate proteoglycan chains normally bind LPL to the capillary endothelium. Heparin, administered as a bolus dose, has a stronger affinity for the LPL binding site than heparan sulfate, leading to the dissociation of heparan-LPL complexes from the endothelium to the plasma. This surge of free LPL is then able to bind to and metabolize chylomicrons and VLDL at an accelerated rate, thus lowering serum TG levels. In case reports, heparin was used in conjunction with an insulin drip or if triglyceride lowering is insufficient despite Nil Per Os (NPO) status, intravenous fluids, and insulin infusions. If heparin is needed despite other interventions, it is safe to start with a standard weight-based infusion to keep the International Normalized Ratio (INR) at 1.5–2 times the upper limit of normal. However, the use of heparin should be limited to short term in order to limit the depletion of LPL stores. There have been numerous reports of the use of heparin and insulin for acute reduction of triglycerides, although there are no established guidelines for efficacy of these modalities, and heparin could possibly be detrimental in the setting of hemorrhagic pancreatitis.

In a nondiabetic patient with severe HTG, a bolus dose of regular insulin (0.1 U/kg) given subcutaneously can decrease serum TG rapidly after a few hours. It has been shown in case reports to be effective either as monotherapy or in conjunction with heparin drip. However, there is insufficient evidence for the benefits of this approach, compared to hemodynamic supportive measures alone.

Evaluate Benefit of Plasmapheresis

Plasmapheresis involves the removal of units of whole blood anti-coagulated with heparin followed by centrifugation to separate the blood into the cellular elements and plasma. The cellular elements are then mixed with a replacement for the discarded plasma and reinfused. Various studies through the years have repeatedly concluded that plasmapheresis is an effective treatment for reducing the serum TG concentration. However, due to the lack of randomized and controlled trials, it is currently unknown if plasmapheresis may improve morbidity and mortality in the clinical setting of HTG-AP. There are currently no consensus clinical guidelines in the management of HTG-AP.

What Is a Safe Therapeutic Target?

An elevated TG level is not a target of therapy per se, to prevent AP, except when very high (>= 500 mg/dL). When TG levels are between 200 and 499 mg/dL, the targets of therapy are non-HDL-C and LDL-C for CV risk reduction. When the TG concentration is very high (>= 500 mg/dL), reducing the concentration to <500 mg/dL to prevent AP becomes the primary goal of therapy. However, some guidelines have concluded that risk of AP decreases if plasma TG concentration is decreased to levels below 1000 mg/dL. Below this level, the treatment goal should be directed toward prevention of premature atherosclerosis.

What Are the Non-pharmacologic Means to Control HTG?

Alcohol consumption should be reduced or eliminated. Lifestyle therapy, including dietary counseling to achieve appropriate diet composition to include foods with low glycemic index, physical activity, and a program to achieve weight reduction in overweight and obese individuals, is recommended as the initial treatment of mild-to-moderate hypertriglyceridemia.

For severe and very severe hypertriglyceridemia (>1000 mg/ dl), combining reduction of total dietary fat and simple carbohydrate intake with prophylactic drug treatment to reduce the risk of AP is recommended. Dietary modification should decrease weight, overall energy intake and intake of all fat (including saturated, unsaturated, and trans fats), and refined carbohydrates. NCEP and NLA advise a carbohydrate intake of 55%–60% and a protein intake of 15%–20% of the daily dietary intake. However, reduction in total fat intake is the cornerstone of treatment for preventing AP and should be limited to less than 15–20% of total calories. Plasma TG response to diet and weight loss is about 25%, with marked variation among patients. Medium-chain triglycerides (MCTs) may be added to make up caloric intake in patients with recurrent AP, as MCTs are not dependent on LPL for hydrolysis.

Determine the Appropriateness of Starting Fibrate Therapy

Treatment with fibrates has been found to be cost-effective as both monotherapy and combination therapy for lowering TG in the prevention of AP. However, the role of fibrates in the prevention of atherosclerotic cardiovascular disease (ASCVD) outcomes in statin-treated patients with optimal LDL-C remains controversial, with some evidence supporting their role in ASCVD event reduction in those with TG concentrations of 200–499 mg/dL and HDL-C concentrations <40 mg/dL. A more potent fibrate, pemafibrate, currently not available, is undergoing a long-term clinical trial for ASCVD event reduction.

Fibrates decrease triglyceride levels by 30–50%. Fibrates may act by multifactorial mechanisms including increased fatty acid oxidation, increased LPL synthesis, reduced expression of Apo CIII, decreased VLDL-TG production, and increased LPL-mediated catabolism of triglyceride-rich lipoproteins (TRL).

Determine Appropriateness of Starting Omega-3-Fatty Acid (OM3FA) Therapy

Use of OM3FAs is an effective TG-lowering treatment option, frequently in combination therapy, in the prevention of AP in high-risk patients with TG levels ≥500 mg/dl.

The long-chain marine OM3FA [eicosapentaenoic acid, C20:5n-3 (EPA), and docosahexaenoic acid, C22:6n-3 (DHA)] can lower fasting and postprandial TG levels in a dose-dependent fashion. Doses of roughly 3–4 g/d of EPA plus DHA are necessary to reduce HTG by 20–40%. OM3FAs are available by prescription in capsules that contain >90% of OM3FA in variable proportion of EPA and DHA. In contrast, over-the-counter preparations of OM3FA have variable quantities of EPA and DHA ranging from 20 to 50%, depending on the products, and generally are not recommended for this purpose.

A recently completed large cardiovascular trial, REDUCE-IT, employed 4 g daily of pure EPA vs placebo in patients with type 2 diabetes, with or without preexisting CVD, with TG 150–499 mg/dl at baseline. All subjects were on statin therapy and optimally controlled LDL-C. In this trial, there was an impressive 25% reduction in major CV end points. However, the CV outcomes were unrelated to the magnitude of TG reduction. This study points to some unique CVD benefits of pure EPA.

Determine Appropriateness of Starting Niacin Therapy

Niacin therapy is recommended principally as an adjunct for reducing TG, if fibrates and OM3FA are not adequately effective. At doses of 500–2000 mg/d, niacin lowers triglycerides by 10–30%, increases HDL cholesterol by 10–40%, and lowers LDL cholesterol by 5–20%. Patients with glucose intolerance and those with DM on oral medications or insulin, who have moderate to good glycemic control, can safely use niacin at moderate dosage, as an adjunct to keep TG in safe range.

However, niacin should not be used for ASCVD event reduction in individuals aggressively treated with a statin due to an absence of evidence for additional CV benefits in those with well-controlled LDL-C (<70–80 mg/dl). In the pre-statin era, high-dose niacin was found to reduce plaque progression in several clinical trials, but given the adverse effects including worsening of glucose control at higher dosage, it is currently not recommended for CVD reduction.

Determine Appropriateness of Starting HMG-CoA Reductase Inhibitors (Statins)

HMG-CoA reductase inhibitors, also known as statins, have a weak TG-lowering effect. They should not be used as monotherapy for HTG. They can have a synergistic TG-lowering effect in combination with fibrates and may be considered in patients in whom HTG is not controlled on fibrates or other TG-lowering agents. In combination therapy of statins with fibrates, fenofibrate is preferred over gemfibrozil, to prevent the risk of myositis.

Evaluate Novel and Potential Therapies of TG-Lowering Agents

Apolipoprotein CIII inhibitors are a novel class of drugs available for patients with familial chylomicronemia syndrome (FCS) for TG reduction. Apolipoprotein CIII (Apo CIII), which is primarily synthesized in the liver, is a key regulator of lipoprotein metabolism and plasma TG levels. It has a role in inhibiting the LPL-mediated hydrolysis of triglyceride-rich lipoproteins (TRL). It also affects the receptor-mediated hepatic uptake of remnants of TRL. It can also inhibit the activity of hepatic lipase at higher concentrations. Apo CIII is an independent risk factor for CVD and is associated with both impaired lipolysis and impaired clearance of TRL from the circulation.

Apo CIII inhibitors are second-generation, single-stranded, DNA-like antisense oligonucleotides designed specifically to bind to a specific RNA sequence. These then elicit degradation of the RNA through RNase H1 and allow the antisense drugs to selectively inhibit Apo CIII synthesis.

Reductions in Apo CIII and TG levels have been reported in a small number of patients with the familial chylomicronemia syndrome who were treated with Apo CIII inhibitors. These patients had defective LPL, and the mechanism of lowering of plasma TG levels was shown to be from an enhanced removal of TRL in a dose-dependent manner. These drugs are currently in phase III studies. Whether targeted reduction of Apo CIII will confer such a benefit in patients at high risk for CVD, including patients with DM and HTG, remains to be determined.

Other novel approaches, in development, to reduce HTG include gene therapy for LPL deficiency and antibody-based therapies.

Acknowledgments OG was partially supported by NIDDK grant # P30-DK036836.

Suggested Readings

Berglund L, Brunzell JD, Goldberg AC, et al. Evaluation and treatment of hypertriglyceridemia: an endocrine society clinical practice guideline. J Clin Endocrinol Metab. 2012;97:2969–89.

Bhatt DL, Steg PG, Miller M, Brinton EA, Jacobson TA, Ketchum SB, et al. REDUCE-IT investigators. Cardiovascular risk reduction with icosapent ethyl for hypertriglyceridemia. N Engl J Med. 2019;380:11–22.

Brahm AJ, Hegele RA. Chylomicronaemia--current diagnosis and future therapies. Nat Rev Endocrinol. 2015;11:352–62.

Chait A, Eckel RH. The Chylomicronemia syndrome is most often multifactorial: a narrative review of causes and treatment of the chylomicronemia syndrome. Ann Intern Med. 2019; https://doi.org/10.7326/M19-0203.

Jacobson TA, Maki KC, Orringer CE, et al. National lipid association recommendations for patient-centered management of dyslipidemia: part 2. J Clin Lipidol. 2015;9:S1–122.

Nakhoda S, Zimrin AB, Baer MR, Law JY. Use of the APACHE II score to assess impact of therapeutic plasma exchange for critically ill patients with hypertriglyceride-induced pancreatitis. Transfus Apher Sci. 2017;56:123–6.

Rocha NA, East C, Zhang J, McCullough PA. ApoCIII as a cardiovascular risk factor and modulation by the novel lipid-lowering agent volane-sorsen. Curr Atheroscler Rep. 2017;19:62.

Scherer J, Singh VP, Pitchumoni CS, Yadav D. Issues in hypertriglyceridemic pancreatitis: an update. J Clin Gastroenterol. 2014;48:195–203.

Hypomagnesemia

29

Alan Ona Malabanan

Contents

A. O. Malabanan (✉)
Beth Israel Deaconess Medical Center, Harvard Medical School,
Division of Endocrinology, Diabetes and Metabolism,
Boston, MA, USA
e-mail: amalaban@bidmc.harvard.edu

© Springer Nature Switzerland AG 2020
R. K. Garg et al. (eds.), *Handbook of Inpatient Endocrinology*,
https://doi.org/10.1007/978-3-030-38976-5_29

Hypomagnesemia Should Be Considered in Patients with Hypocalcemia or Hypokalemia, Cardiac Dysrhythmias (Torsades de Pointes), Alcoholism, Diabetes, Diarrheal Illnesses, Renal Tubular Disorders and Use of Medications Associated with Hypomagnesemia such as Proton Pump Inhibitors, Diuretics, Cisplatin, and Amphotericin B

Magnesium is an important intracellular cofactor for a multitude of cellular processes, and deficiency can disrupt several organ systems. The human body has approximately 25 g of magnesium, 50–60% of which is found in the bone. Magnesium homeostasis is maintained by balancing dietary magnesium absorption and urinary magnesium losses. Up to 60–70% of a dietary magnesium load is absorbed in the gut, the majority in the ileum, with its absorption aided by high gastric acidity. Intestinal magnesium absorption is not regulated. Diarrheal illnesses cause increased magnesium losses and disrupt intestinal magnesium absorption. Serum magnesium levels are controlled primarily through reabsorption by the kidneys. Illnesses or medications causing diuresis, such as alcoholism, diabetes mellitus or insipidus, or diuretics, lead to increased urinary losses of magnesium. Proton pump inhibitors decrease intestinal magnesium absorption. Cisplatin and amphotericin B may cause renal tubular dysfunction leading to urinary magnesium losses. Magnesium is important for parathyroid hormone release and action, which can disrupt calcium homeostasis. In addition, it is a cofactor for the sodium-potassium ATPase, and deficiency leads to hypokalemia. As such, hypomagnesemia may cause neuromuscular and cardiac irritability.

Serum Magnesium Does Not Reflect Total Body Magnesium Stores and a Total Body Magnesium Deficit May Exist Even with a Normal Serum Magnesium Level

Extracellular magnesium represents only 1% of the total body magnesium. As a result, serum magnesium is not an accurate measure of total body magnesium stores and cannot accurately demonstrate successful repletion of body magnesium stores. A test for red blood cell magnesium is available, but due to prolonged turnaround time as well as artifact related to improper specimen processing, it is of limited utility in the inpatient setting. Magnesium treatment should be considered, even with a normal serum magnesium level, if there is hypocalcemia, hypokalemia, or drugs/conditions associated with hypomagnesemia.

A 24-Hour Urine Magnesium and Creatinine or a Fractional Excretion of Magnesium May Be Useful in Establishing the Etiology of Hypomagnesemia

Body magnesium is controlled by a balance between gastrointestinal magnesium absorption, skeletal magnesium storage, and urinary magnesium losses. Most cellular food (i.e., of animal or plant origin) have significant amounts of magnesium, which are typically readily absorbed, although there are concerns of decreasing magnesium content of the Western diet. Gastrointestinal dysfunction, either with increased motility leading to diarrhea or problems with absorption such as inflammatory bowel disease, will lead to decreased magnesium absorption. A daily 24-hour urine magnesium excretion, in the setting of hypomagnesemia, of more than 10–30 mg or a fractional excretion of magnesium ($FEMg = ((UMg \times PCr)/(0.7 \times PMg \times UCr)) \times 100\%$) of >2% argues for renal magnesium wasting. A daily 24-hour urine magnesium excretion, in the setting of hypomagnesemia, of <10 mg or an FEMg <2% argues for gastrointestinal losses.

A 24-Hour Urine Magnesium and Creatinine May Be Useful in Confirming Adequacy of Total Body Magnesium Stores

Magnesium sufficiency will lead to increased urinary magnesium losses. Diuresis, either from drugs or conditions, will lead to increased magnesium ultrafiltration and decreased reabsorption of magnesium. Hungry bone syndrome, after parathyroidectomy, will increase the bone uptake of magnesium, as well as calcium and phosphate. The normal physiologic response to hypomagnesemia is an increase in renal reabsorption of magnesium, so an inappropriately normal or high urinary magnesium points to a renal etiology of the hypomagnesemia. In addition, assessing a 24-hour urine magnesium after an intravenous magnesium bolus is helpful. A high 24-hour urine magnesium excretion indicates magnesium sufficiency, although this assessment is not typically practical in most hospitalized patients.

Hypocalcemia or Hypokalemia with Concomitant Hypomagnesemia Will Not Correct with Calcium or Potassium Therapy Alone

Magnesium is an important cofactor for the Na-K ATPase and is also important for parathyroid hormone release and action. Persistent or recurrent hypokalemia or hypocalcemia is frequently associated with magnesium deficiency, and consideration of magnesium repletion should be pursued even in the presence of normal serum magnesium.

A Concomitant Assessment of Urinary Calcium Can Help Identify the Portion of the Nephron Affected in Hypomagnesemia

Conditions affecting the loop of Henle, such as loop diuretic use, Bartter's syndrome, or nephrotoxins, will cause hypercalciuria in the setting of hypermagnesiuria. Conditions affecting the early distal nephron, such as Gitelman's syndrome, are associated with hypocalciuria with hypermagnesiuria. Normocalciuria and hypermagnesiuria (i.e., isolated magnesiuria) may be seen in mutations of the pro-epidermal growth factor (pro-EGF) gene or as a result of cetuximab therapy.

Severe Hypomagnesemia (Mg <1 meq/L) and Symptomatic Hypomagnesemia Should Be Treated with Intravenous Magnesium Therapy

The presence of torsades de pointes should be treated emergently with 1–2 g of IV magnesium sulfate over 30–60 seconds. It may be repeated in 5–15 minutes if the arrhythmia does not resolve. For asymptomatic severe hypomagnesemia, 1–2 g of IV magnesium sulfate may be given over 3–6 hours. For both situations, continuous IV magnesium sulfate infusion should be ordered (4–8 g magnesium sulfate over 12–24 hours in those with normal renal function and 50% dose reduction if chronic kidney disease).

Oral Magnesium Oxide Therapy Is Limited by Diarrhea and Often Intravenous Magnesium Sulfate Therapy Is Necessary

Oral magnesium acts as a laxative and at higher doses can cause diarrhea. Oral magnesium can be tried, at small doses (i.e., 250 mg), as tolerated. Small doses every few hours are much better tolerated than larger doses at one time. If the oral magnesium is not tolerated or there is already diarrhea, intravenous magnesium sulfate should be considered. Symptomatic hypomagnesemia, i.e., neuromuscular irritability or cardiovascular dysrhythmias, should be treated urgently with intravenous magnesium sulfate. An ongoing intravenous magnesium sulfate drip should be considered in patients with normal renal function to help replete depleted intracellular magnesium. Table 29.1 shows magnesium preparations and elemental magnesium content.

In Addition to Replacement Magnesium Therapy, Addressing the Etiology of the Hypomagnesemia Is Necessary to Maintain Magnesium Homeostasis

The causes of hypomagnesemia are listed in Table 29.2 and involve either inadequate magnesium intake or absorption or excessive urinary magnesium losses. Assuring adequate intake

Table 29.1 Magnesium preparations

Preparation	Route of administration	% Elemental magnesium	mg/mEq
Magnesium sulfate (1 gm)	IV	10%	100 mg/8.1 mEq
Magnesium chloride (535 mg)	PO	12%	64 mg/5.33 mEq
Magnesium oxide (400 mg)	PO	60%	241.3 mg/20.1 mEq
Magnesium gluconate (500 mg)	PO	5.4%	27 mg/2.25 mEq
Magnesium hydroxide (1200 mg/15 mL)	PO	42%	500 mg/41 mEq
Magnesium citrate (1.745 g/30 mL)	PO	16%	279 mg/23 mEq
Magnesium lactate (Mag-Tab SR caplet)	PO	12%	84 mg/7 mEq
Magnesium L-aspartate (615 mg)	PO	9.9%	61 mg/5 mEq

of magnesium and treating diarrhea is important. If the small intestine has been resected, a parenteral source of magnesium may be necessary. Proton pump inhibitor therapy may need to be discontinued and an alternative acid-lowering therapy substituted.

Table 29.2 Causes of hypomagnesemia

Inadequate intake	Excessive urinary losses	Redistribution
Malnutrition	Drugs	Ethanol withdrawal
Inadequate absorption	Diuretics	Insulin administration
Diarrhea	Aminoglycosides	Hungry bone syndrome
Short bowel syndrome	Cisplatin (Platinol-AQ)	Pancreatitis
Celiac disease	Amphotericin B (Fungizone)	Trisodium phosphonoformate (Foscarnet)
Inflammatory bowel disease	Tacrolimus (Prograf)	Blood transfusion in liver transplant recipients
Laxative abuse	Cyclosporine (Sandimmune)	
Drugs	Cetuximab (Erbitux)	
Proton pump inhibitors	Pentamidine (Nebupent)	
Genetic	Primary tubular disorder	
Primary familial hypomagnesemia	Primary renal wasting	
	Renal tubular acidosis	
	Diuretic phase of acute tubular necrosis	
	Post-obstructive diuresis	
	Post renal transplantation	

(continued)

Table 29.2 (continued)

Inadequate intake	Excessive urinary losses	Redistribution
	Hormone-induced	
	Aldosteronism	
	Hypoparathyroidism and Hyperparathyroidism	
	Hyperthyroidism	
	Genetic	
	Gitelman's syndrome	
	Autosomal dominant hypercalciuric hypocalcemia	
	Miscellaneous (Na-K-ATPase, HNF1B, KCNA1, EGF)	
	Induced tubular losses	
	Hypercalcemia	
	Volume expansion	
	Glucose, urea, mannitol diuresis	
	Phosphate depletion	
	Alcohol ingestion	

Suggested Readings

Agus ZS. Mechanisms and causes of hypomagnesemia. Curr Opin Nephrol Hypertens. 2016;25:301–7.

Ayuk J, Gittoes NJL. Treatment of hypomagnesemia. Am J Kidney Dis. 2014;63:691–5.

de Baaij JHF, Hoenderop JGJ, Bindels RJM. Magnesium in man: implications for health and disease. Physiol Rev. 2015;95:1–46.

Guerrera MP, Volpe SL, Mao JJ. Therapeutic uses of magnesium. Am Fam Physician. 2009;80:157–62.

Ismail Y, Ismail AA, Ismail AAA. The underestimated problem of using serum magnesium measurements to exclude magnesium deficiency in adults; a health warning is needed for "normal" results. Clin Chem Lab Med. 2010;48:323–7.

Index

© Springer Nature Switzerland AG 2020
R. K. Garg et al. (eds.), *Handbook of Inpatient Endocrinology*,
https://doi.org/10.1007/978-3-030-38976-5